A Pain Doctor's Dilemma
Prescribing Opioids in an Era of Overdose

Dr. Richard Ng

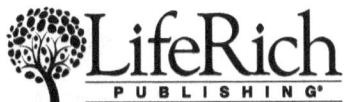
LifeRich
PUBLISHING

LifeRich Publishing is a registered trademark of The Reader's Digest Association, Inc.

LifeRich Publishing books may be ordered through booksellers or by contacting:

LifeRich Publishing
1663 Liberty Drive
Bloomington, IN 47403
www.liferichpublishing.com
1 (888) 238-8637

ISBN: 978-1-4897-1266-0 (sc)
ISBN: 978-1-4897-1267-7 (hc)
ISBN: 978-1-4897-1265-3 (e)

Library of Congress Control Number: 2017907548

Print information available on the last page.

LifeRich Publishing rev. date: 05/16/2017

"For all the happiness mankind can gain,
Is not in pleasure, but in rest from pain."

___ John Dryden (1631 – 1700)

Acknowledgement

I would not have survived my five years of uncertainty, stress, mental anguish, personal crises, near poverty, vicissitude and depression without the love and kindness, unwavering trust, financial support, and countless hours of legal research of my brother-in-law and attorney, Steve Bonnette, and his wife, Ruth Hoi-Tak Bonnette, who is my youngest sister in a family of eleven children.

Contents

Foreword

Pain does not discriminate. It can happen to the young and old, rich and poor, men and women, the healthy and sick; it can also happen to the educated people with good jobs, and to those performing menial work. Nobody is exempt from pain, and you will experience it sooner or later. Pain affects people differently with vast individual variations. For some people, their pain requires immediate relief; others will try to tough it out, hoping that the pain will go away. There are some pain sufferers who believe that pain is the wrath from God or some supreme beings as punishment for their transgressions, and these believers will resist and refuse any intervention for their pain.

Regardless of your circumstances or personal belief, ignoring your pain can be dangerous with serious consequences. If the pain is left untreated, or is under-treated, it can have profound, deleterious effects on your well-being, both physically and mentally.

There are many different methods of treatment for chronic pain, as discussed in chapter nine of this book. People suffering from chronic pain usually have tried many treatment modalities without satisfactory results before they go to the pain doctors for opioid painkillers, which are effective for pain management. Unfortunately, due to a very small subgroup of pain patients who have become addicted to opioids while receiving prescriptions for controlled substances for their pain, the medical management of chronic, non-cancer pain with opioids has become controversial. The situation is made worse with the rising number of overdoses, some lethal, in the past decade in the United States. In many other countries, patients are typically held more accountable for problems related to opioid prescriptions written by physicians with proper dosages and instruction.

In the United States, there seems to be a trend to place the blame for the so-called crisis of opioid overdose on the prescribing doctors. This has already created problematic issues on many fronts. The truth is: people with addictive behaviors will and can find what they want anywhere and continue to exacerbate the ' war on drugs ', while millions of legitimate patients with chronic pain continue to suffer with compromised functionality, poor quality of life and mental health, and decreased productivity in our American society. This is the real public health crisis!

Chapter One

What is pain?

At the turn of this century, the Congress of the United States designated it as the Decade of Pain Awareness. It is undeniable and a statistical fact that controlled substance prescriptions for pain have increased many folds since the beginning of the 21st century. More and more patients are open enough to discuss about their pain with their doctors. The general and family practitioners are still the primary providers that deal with most of the patients with chronic pain. Even though there are more physicians specialized in pain management, their number is still comparatively small while the number of patients with chronic pain is increasing every day.

According to the National Institute of Neurological Disorders and Stroke, more than 100 million Americans experience some form of pain that lasts from a few days to a few weeks and to even years. Moreover, everyone will suffer from some type of pain temporarily, whether due to a headache, an infected tooth, an abrasion or a cut on the skin, or a broken bone. While it is easy to just think of " pain is pain ", the reality is far more complex because everyone deals with pain differently.

What is pain? Pain, as defined by the International Association for the Study of Pain, is an unpleasant sensory and emotional experience associated with actual or potential tissue damage. While you can easily tell when some part of your body physically hurts, your pain cannot be objectively assessed or measured by others because only you know precisely what hurts, how badly and what that pain feels like. Simply put, pain is, therefore, whatever the person experiencing it says it is.

The origin of the word ' pain ' is Latin and derived from the word ' peona ' which means suffering, punishment and penalty. Pain is very private and personal, and to know whether a person is experiencing pain, it must be made public through verbal, or non-verbal signals or behaviors.

Some people call pain the fifth vital sign, along with blood pressure, temperature, pulse rate and respiratory rate. Ironically, we can exactly measure the first four of the vital signs, but the amount or level of pain still cannot be measured objectively. Pain as the 5th vital sign was a Veterans Administration initiative born in the late 1990s.

However, pain can be divided into two categories:

Acute pain: it typically comes on suddenly due to some injury, disease, illness, infection or inflammation, and the cause can usually be determined and treated. While an acute pain can sometimes evoke feelings of fear, anxiety and/or restlessness in the person, the pain and any physical or emotional symptoms generally subside within a few hours, days or weeks with appropriate treatments. If the underlying cause of the acute pain cannot be correctly diagnosed and effectively treated, an acute pain can develop into a chronic pain.

Chronic pain: it can be mild, moderate, severe or intractable., and it may last for a long time --- for six months of more up to many years including a lifetime. The persistence of chronic pain can be very debilitating, and in severe cases, can lead to other issues such as feelings of depression, social withdrawal, physical and emotional exhaustion as well as the loss of mobility and/or independence. The worst case scenario is suicide, which is not uncommon among patients suffering from chronic pain.

Some people get chronic pain from normal wear and tear of the body or from aging. Every person is different and perceives and experiences pain in different ways. There is often very little consistency when different doctors try to measure a patient's pain. Sometimes, the doctor may not believe the patient, or might minimize the amount of pain. All of these things can be frustrating for the person in pain. In some cases, the chronic pain may be from an injury that happened during an accident or an assault. Truthfully, some chronic pain has no explanation.

This book is written for brave and compassionate doctors in pain management with opioid, for patients suffering from chronic pain, and the general public to promote understanding, awareness and education.

Our pain is mediated by our Central Nervous System (CNS) which consists of the brain and the spinal cord.

A huge network of nerves (the Peripheral Nervous System) extends from the spinal cord into different parts of the body such as skin, muscles and internal organs. When some sort of bodily injury occurs, such as cutting your finger while peeling an apple with a knife, pain receptors called nociceptors send signals along the peripheral nerves in your finger to the spinal cord, which then transmits this message to certain specific areas of the brain.

The nociceptors in your body detect injuries which can fall into two types:

Somatic pain: this refers to pain from traumas to your bones, joints or soft tissues including muscles and skin. Somatic pain is usually localized, meaning the location can be easily verified, and it is often described as sharp, dull aching or throbbing. Common examples of somatic pain include bone fractures and arthritis.

Visceral pain: it results when the nociceptors detect inflammation, distension or stretching or our internal organs. This type of pain is generally not localized, and often described as cramping, deep or pressure-type. Examples of visceral pain include appendicitis, abdominal pain from bowel obstruction, and pain in the left arm, left shoulder and/or jaw from a heart attack (myocardial infarction).

Chronic pain becomes chronic when pain does not go away after the normal healing time allowed. There is some variation in terms of the required pain duration, in that some conditions may become chronic in as little as one month, while some pain specialists adhere to the six-month pain duration criteria. Anyone that suffers with a chronic pain condition knows well that it not only affects the body, but also the mind. Sometimes, its effect on a sufferer's mind can almost be worse than the pain itself. Many health care providers fail to recognize the complexity of pain and simply believe that it can be dichotomized based on the presence or absence of physical findings, secondary gain, or prior emotional problems. As a result, so many patients have been informed that " The pain is all in your head ". And if these same patients react with anger and hurt, we (the health care providers and staff) are ready to compound the problem by labeling them as hostile, demanding, or aggressive.

In actuality, the correspondence between physical, objective findings such as MRI, CT, or X-ray results and pain complaints is fairly low, generally 40% to 60%. Patients may have abnormal tests showing a bulging disc or a herniation with no or negligible pain, or substantial pain with seemingly negative test results. This is because chronic pain can develop in the absence of gross abnormal changes we are able to detect with current technology. Muscle strain and inflammation are common causes of chronic pain, yet may be very difficult to detect. There are other painful conditions due to systemic problems such as HIV-related pain or sickle cell pain, trauma to nerves such as post-thoracotomy pain, circulatory issues such as diabetic neuropathy, or many others. In each of these cases, we may not be able to ' see ' the cause of the pain problem, instead, we have to rely on the patient's report of their pain, coupled with behavioral observations and some available indirect medical data. This does not mean that the pain is psychogenic. Rather, it means that we are unable to detect or understand its cause.

There are quite a few factors that can influence the experience of pain, and let us look at some of them:

- Site of injury
- Degree of tissue damage
- Density of receptors present
- Intensity of stimulation
- Emotional status of the individual
- Attentional effects
- General health of the person with pain
- The individual's belief regarding their ability to deal with the pain
- The individual's expectations because pain can be experienced without noxious stimulation if it is expected.
- The person's history of pain experiences.

Pain is often considered as a symptom, but over time, chronic pain may develop into what we call the "Chronic Pain Syndrome" exhibiting some or many of the symptoms as follows:

- Decreased activity
- Disrupted sleep
- Irritability
- Fatigue
- Impaired memory and cognitive function
- Low self-esteem
- Difficulty in sexual relationship due to lack of interest
- Kinesiophobia, which is the avoidance of certain movements or activities due to fear of re-injury
- Anxiety
- Poor performance at work, leading to loss of job
- Difficulty interacting and raising children at home
- Poor house-keeping
- Alcohol abuse
- Medication abuse
- Feeling of helplessness
- Feeling of hopelessness
- Guilt

- Depression
- Social isolation

With the last four or five symptoms above, it is not surprising that individuals suffering from chronic, intractable pain may have suicidal ideation and/or attempt.

It is estimated that about 30% of the U.S. population suffers with chronic pain. Pain can bring about different physical symptoms like nausea, dizziness, weakness or drowsiness. It can also cause emotional effects such as anger, depression, mood swings or irritability. Perhaps most significantly, it can change your lifestyle and impact your job, relationships and independence.

Being in pain is quite uncomfortable for most of us; for the very few people who are lucky enough to never experience any pain, I am very happy for them. Even minor pain such as a paper cut is unpleasant but that pain fades quickly. Imagine being in pain that never goes away, or that fades only to come back in a few hours later. What would that do to a person? This is what people with chronic pain have to deal with every day.

Chronic pain can be brought on by a wide range of illnesses, including cancers, low back disorders, arthritis and degenerative joint diseases, shingles, fibromyalgia, sickle cell anemia, diabetic neuropathy, HIV/AIDS, migraine and cluster headaches, fractures, sports injuries, motor vehicle accidents, and post-surgical pain.

Chronic pain can have a profound effect on a person's day-to-day life when it goes untreated and under-treated. Constant, chronic pain raises the focus threshold for basic functioning, which leaves the suffering person with a greatly reduced ability to find solutions to even relatively mundane things. Something like a traffic jam, which most people would be annoyed by but ultimately take in stride, could easily and seriously throw off the rhythm of someone in pain, putting forth so much effort just to get through the day.

Chronic pain, including its intractable form, wears a person down, draining their energy and lessening their motivation. Patients with chronic pain sometimes will try to limit social contacts in an effort to reduce and reduce the amount of energy they have to spend reacting to their surroundings. As a result, many people with chronic pain, roughly one third of them, develop depression at some point during their lifetime, with symptoms such as anxiety, lack of interpersonal interactions, difficulty concentrating on even simple tasks, and seeking isolation and quiet, and feeling of hopelessness, which can lead to suicidal ideation and attempt.

Speaking of suicidal thoughts and attempt, I remembered three patients of mine; two had history of suicidal attempts and one had suicidal ideation off and on because their pain was hard to control despite dosages above the recommended therapeutic ranges. I had tried to refer them to counseling centers like Sinnissippi Center in Dixon, Illinois, for mental health treatment. Because they were self-pay without any insurance coverage, they were given appointments in 60 days. I was told that they should go to the ER for any urgent need.

I spent additional time for these three patients with counseling in my office even though I was not a certified therapist. Psychology was my second major in college. When I was a medical student, I had a psychiatry clinical rotation for four weeks at VA Hines Hospital in Maywood, Illinois. In my private pain practice, I also had quite a few CME hours in addiction.

I was glad that I was able to help the patients out as much as I could. I vividly recalled telling them that suicide did not end the suffering of pain; it passed onto their survivors and loved ones.

Sleeping seems to make the pain less intrusive, and that combined with the exhaustion from the pain means that it is rather common for a pain patient to try to sleep upwards of ten hours a day. Despite the amount of sleep or rest, patients with chronic pain do not feel the energy or motivation like the normal people with sufficient sleep.

Some studies have shown that chronic pain can actually affect a person's brain chemistry and even change the wiring of the nervous system. Cells in the spinal cord and the brain of a person with chronic pain seem to deteriorate more quickly than normal, and can create biologically a feeling of hopelessness. Making it more difficult to process future pain in a healthy way. Untreated and under-treated chronic pain creates a downward spiral; one thing is clear, however, the earlier a person receives effective treatment, the less the pain will affect their day-to-day life.

Treating pain with opioids will inherently cause tolerance and physical dependence, which many people confuse them with addiction. Only a very small percentage of patients exposed to opioids will develop addiction and this phenomenon is rather unpredictable. Whereas, the repeated administration of any opioid will inevitably lead to the development of tolerance and physical dependence. These predictable phenomena and short-term results of repeated opioid administration will resolve rapidly after discontinuation of the opioids, anywhere from a few days to a few weeks, depending on the duration of exposure, dosage and type of opioids. The molecular processes responsible for addiction are distinct from those underlying tolerance and physical dependence, and so are the clinical consequences.

With repeated exposure to the opioid, its potency will decrease due to the phenomenon of tolerance. Thus, prescribing opioids for long-term pain management will typically require increasingly higher doses in order to attain the initial level of analgesia, sometimes, up to ten times the original dose. In general, tolerance usually develops slowly, in contrast, euphoric effects of opioid develops quickly. Insidiously, tolerance to respiratory depression by opioid also develops slowly, which explains why increases in dose by the prescriber or patient to maintain analgesia can increase the risk of overdose.

Physical dependence underlies the physiological adaptations that are responsible for the manifestation of withdrawal symptoms upon abrupt discontinuation of the opioid. The symptoms of withdrawal include restlessness, pilo-erection, shaking chills, insomnia, nausea, diarrhea, vomiting and muscle aches. They vary in severity (from mildly noticeable to very uncomfortable and distressful) and duration (from one to fourteen days) on the basis of the type, dose and duration of opioid prescribed.

Chapter Two

Pseudo-addiction and addiction

The understanding of addiction and pain has come a long way, and there is still a lot of work ahead of us for the treatments of patients with chronic and intractable pain, including terminology and biologic concepts.

The famous pioneer, Howard Hughes, makes an interesting case for the discussion of addiction and pseudo-addiction. Unfortunately and mistakenly, some people called him an addict with a reclusive and addictive personality. Born in 1905, he was a unique, world-recognized entrepreneur engaged in diverse ventures that included chemicals, plastics, motion pictures, entertainment, aircraft design and development.

In 1946, the 41 year-old intelligent man survived a serious crash in in the aircraft he designed and developed with multiple major injuries. His pain-producing injuries included third-degree burn of abdomen, chest wall, face and extremities. He also sustained multiple fractures including the facial area, multiple fractures of ribs bilaterally, fracture of the left clavicle and fractures of the $5^{th}, 6^{th}$ and 7th cervical vertebrae. He was hospitalized at Good Samaritan Hospital in the city of Los Angeles for about five weeks with morphine for pain, and was discharged on codeine.

Modern day pain management clearly recognizes that his

injuries are very likely, if not certainly, associated with intractable pain, a term that was not used during the life of Hughes. Intractable pain refers to the more severe form of chronic pain, which is incapacitating, constant, incurable, and interfering with multiple biologic functions such as sleep, eating, ambulation, social interactions and mental health issues. Under-treatment results in reclusiveness, home or bed-bound state, and sometimes, suicide. Analysis of Hughes' medical and pain history definitely shows that today he would be characterized as an intractable-pain patient.

The degenerative arthritis in many joints as he aged must have aggravated his pain. He also had allodynia, which presents as severe pain to the touch. At times, his pain was reported to be so severe that a simple touch or the touching of bed-linens or pyjamas produced unbearable pain. Because he had taken high doses of codeine and diazepam for many years, he was wrongly labeled an addict by many concerned parties.

Today, Hughes' drug seeking would be termed pseudo-addiction, a term which was not understood or used until 1980. There is now a standard set of terms adopted by all major professional pain treatment organizations and the American Society of Addiction Medicine.

Hughes, with his doctor's instruction, self-injected pure codeine phosphate and also took oral compounded codeine with phenacetin and aspirin. It is now clear that codeine would not be potent enough or last long enough in the body or provide much pain relief for Hughes when he required pain relief 24 hours a day. In his defense posthumously, Hughes did not have the usual addictive personality witnessed in today's America. He did not smoke cigarettes and seldom drank alcohol even with his busy social lifestyle before his plane crash. He did not routinely inject codeine by the intravenously as would an addict but, instead, he injected it into the subcutaneous and muscular tissues.

The activity log kept by his aides between 1971 and 1973 revealed that he had taken 8 to 10 codeine (480mg to 600mg) at one time indicating considerable tolerance and longtime use of codeine. About 10mg of codeine are equivalent to 1mg of morphine, so Hughes was taking the equivalence of 140mg to 270mg of morphine a day. This is considered a low to moderate dose for many of today's intractable pain patients. Today, it is not uncommon for the daily morphine dosage to exceed 1000mg a day.

With careful investigation, Hughes probably received inadequate pain relief from codeine, and he suffered severe complications from under-treatment of chronic pain. Due to codeine's weak pain relief and numerous complications, it is essentially not used today for intractable pain syndrome.

During the wars on drugs in the 1980's and 1990's, our government agents, both federal and local, risked their lives going after drug gangs on the streets. They arrested hundreds of thousands of people annually and filled majority of American prison cells with drug offenders. However, drugs remained as available as ever on the streets – and actually got a lot cheaper and more potent and deadly. With the rising number of lethal drug overdoses, even though most of them had taken other drugs and medications, the search for blame has been shifted to doctors and clinics, pharmaceutical wholesalers and pharmacies. The trendy and common diagnosis on the death certificate for the cause of death is poly-pharmacy, which is actually misleading and convenient.

Physicians offered several advantages over crack, meth and heroin dealers. Doctors are not armed. They are listed in the telephone books. They can be spotted easily online. They keep office hours and records of their transactions. And unlike the typical, dangerous drug dealers living with their mothers or hard-to-find places, doctors usually have valuable assets that can be seized and shared by the federal, state and local agencies fighting the so-called drug war. Apart from the uncertainty of the cause of death in these cases, many figures released by different governmental agencies have been exaggerated as compared with the higher number of people who died from gastrointestinal bleeding and related complications from other painkillers, like ibuprofen, aspirin, naproxen and acetaminophen.

The current zeal for sending doctors to jail for writing painkiller prescriptions may seem baffling. Especially to the patients who rely on the doctors for pain relief. While it is true that chronic-pain patients taking opioids for a long time will require higher and higher doses, the drug typically don't give them a high or interfere with their lives. Instead, the prescribed drugs enable them to function with quality of life. This is NOT addiction!

Researchers have repeatedly found that very few patients taking opioids for chronic pain have a hard time stopping once their pain goes away. The ones who can't stop – the compulsive addicts – are typically people with a history of abusing alcohol and other drugs

More and more doctors are now afraid to give painkillers to patients who truly need them for relief. There are many doctors who label their patients unfairly, demean their patients and degrade them because they are victims of chronic life-long pain. This is archaic medicine and does more harm than one can imagine: physicians are afraid to treat patients with the diagnosis of chronic pain, even from legitimate conditions.

Sometimes, physicians are unable to find the clear cause for their patients' pain, but that is not to say the pain does not exist. It is understandable that physicians and other healthcare providers may become frustrated due to diagnostic dilemma. With the current atmosphere of suspicion and fear, many patients with chronic pain are being sent away with plausible excuses, smacking of abandonment. Once a pain patient is refused treatment or discharged by a physician, in such circumstances, he or she would run into insurmountable difficulty getting accepted by anyone else in the medical community.

Since doctors who prescribe narcotic pain medications have become targets of scrutiny by local pharmacists and investigation by the Government, more and more of them are afraid and refusing to treat patients with chronic pain. Pain patients are far too often considered malingering or doctor shopping. They are being labeled as long-term drug users by physicians, nurses and government authorities with very negative implications. This prejudicial, unfair treatment often causes far-reaching damage, both physically and mentally. It has adverse effect on family, friends and co-workers, and often causes the pain sufferers to withdraw from society, including normal daily activities with their spouses, friends and family.

Much like the abortion issue, many patients with chronic pain are being forced into back alleyways, store front pain clinic and worse. This kind of sad and unfair treatment forces them into seeking help and relief outside of the Law. They rarely receive counseling on how to take their medications and many don't even know what they are taking. It is one issue to target and stamp out illegal or unscrupulous clinics doling out prescriptions for pain pills without even carefully examining the patients, but another issue entirely to target physicians with well intention. I am not saying that there are no bad physicians; but they represent a miniscule of the medical community, a few black sheep on the huge pasture.

To make the matter worse for patients with chronic pain, pharmacists often feel the need to interfere and embarrass the patients when they turn in or pick up their pain medications. I understand that they should be careful and vigilant dealing with controlled substances, many of them have become so judgmental due to pressure from the Authority that they are treating the pain patients like second or third-class citizens.

A large study was conducted at the Anderson Cancer Center in Houston, Texas, looking at more than 3,000 patients suffering pain from invasive cancers of the breast, prostate, lung, colon and rectum. Researchers found that at least one-third of the patients were prescribed inadequate medications to control the pain they were experiencing. Surprisingly, the treating physicians of these suffering patients in the study were aware of the problems of under-treatment of pain. Isn't this ironical and unconscionable? Another problem that doctors face is objectively determining how much pain a patient is actually experiencing. The most commonly asked question --- ' what is your pain on the scale of one to ten? ' --- often does not paint a complete picture, according to the researchers.

Society's negative view of certain types of pain medications seem to have created a major problem. The fear of overdose, potential abuse and over-use, and addiction can make a doctor very hesitant to prescribe the appropriate pain medicine and the appropriate dosages for patients. The current environment is more concerned about the illegal use of controlled substances than the appropriate use.

As reported by ABC Medical Unit in 2012, 60 years old Johnie Bennett of Newhall, California was diagnosed with lung cancer. The diagnosis not only threatened her life, it also kept her in constant pain. " It does become tedious ", she said of her efforts to control her pain. " It becomes a job, one that you resent ". While her pain was considerable and sometimes unbearable, she said that she hesitated to use the pain medications all the time for fear of becoming addicted.

Bennett's story is common among pain-suffering patients. As many as one third of cancer patients may be receiving inadequate treatment to control their pain, even though many effective medicines are approved by our Government and available to help, many researches suggest. Many patients in my practice with documented diagnoses such as herniated discs of the cervical and lumbar spine, failed back surgery syndrome, degenerative disc disease, sciatica, advanced arthritis and so on were often treated with disrespect, suspicion and sometimes disdain, causing unnecessary and additional anguish and emotional pain.

Pain receptors can malfunction, and injuries can cause pain years later. Elderly patients who suffer chronic pain every remaining day of their life are told by their doctors that they are concerned about possible addiction, even though the percentage of patients taking controlled substances for pain is very low, according to many studies. What happened to the quality of their life? Their right to live their life without debilitating pain? Their only option may be to consider suicide? In fact, the high suicide rate among patients with chronic pain is almost deliberately ignored and rarely discussed.

The new class of physicians from medical schools are taught that any patient requesting pain medications is to be suspected and scrutinized; what about the importance of the history and self-reporting of complaints in the H & P? We are ironically graduating a class of new doctors on how NOT to treat patients with pain --- this is a horror!

If enough doctors are jailed or scared into not writing pain prescriptions, it is conceivable that this war on drug could have more impact than the ones against heroin and cocaine – doctors, after all, are harder to replace than crack and heroin dealers. But even if there is less NORCO and OxyContin on the streets, is this worth the suffering of so many patients who can't get the legal painkillers they need? Because the diverted OxyContin and NORCO are more expensive and difficult to purchase, users have switched to heroin resulting in the rising number of heroin overdoses, according to Government reports.

There has been a literature consensus reached on the need for chronic opioid treatment for patients with chronic pain if other treatments fail, but there is a subpopulation within the group that is problematic. Other evidence also indicates that majority of the patients with chronic pain can achieve sustained satisfactory analgesia from opioid therapy without the occurrence of intolerable side effects. Impairment of daily activity, psychomotor speed, and sustained attention and mood have also been reported to improve with long-term opioid treatment for them.

We need to make the distinction between addiction and pseudo-addiction because they are not the same, even though some of the behaviors may overlap. Once the pain is controlled with appropriate medications and adequate dosages, the questionable behaviors disappear. Because many pain patients may not have the access to proper care, they may exhibit behavior that may be construed as the actions of an addict.

It is puzzling and incredible why so many people are so

judgmental and assuming. Who would not want the pain to stop? It is unreasonable for anyone to suffer with pain; the pain medication is there for a reason. It may look scary to the doctors, family, friends, colleagues and co-workers when a pain sufferer is desperate to ensure access to medications. It is disturbing to watch someone you love be counting down the days to a renewal of prescriptions. However, the behavior must be understood by everyone. As far as I know from my years of pain practice, none of the patients with chronic pain is happy about taking the pain medications, except for a few problematic ones which I eventually discharged after repeated warnings. Nor do they feel a euphoria or ' high ' sensation when they are taking the medications. They simply want relief from the pain.

Untreated and undertreated chronic pain is not only an epidemic, it's a crime. According to a stunning news report by Human Rights Watch (HRW), the majority of the world's population lacks adequate access to narcotic pain relief. . Governments are letting their own people suffer needlessly and flouting international law in the process. In signing the 1961 Single Convention on Narcotic Drugs, the international community acknowledged that narcotic drugs are indispensable for the relief of pain and suffering, and signatories from different countries were committed to making these drugs available to those in need. However, HRW reports that most nations are failing to live up to that commitment. Eighty percent of the world's population currently have inadequate access to opioid painkillers.

HRW further reports that "the poor availability of pain treatment is both perplexing and inexcusable. Pain causes terrible suffering yet the medications to treat it are cheap, effective, and safe with proper monitoring, and generally straightforward to administer. Over the last twenty years, the World Health Organization (WHO) and the International Narcotics Council Board (INCB), the body that monitors the implementation of the U.N. drug conventions have repeatedly reminded nations of their obligations. But little progress has been made in many countries.

The HRW report blames government inaction and excessively strict drug control policies for the prevalent practice of untreated and under-treated pain. Many governments are so afraid that narcotics will be diverted for illicit purposes that they are willing to let sick people go without in order to keep criminals from cashing in. This warped logic is the equivalent of imprisoning the innocent to make sure that the guilty don't go free. Cultural and legal barriers get in the way of good pain medicine. Unfortunately and understandably, physicians are afraid of narcotics, like the low-information general population. Doctors in Kenya are so used to patients dying in pain that they think this is how you must die. The palliative care movement has made some inroads in the West, but pharmacological puritanism and overblown concerns about addiction and overdoses are still major barriers to pain relief. In the U.S., many doctors hesitate to prescribe narcotic painkillers according to their medical training their conscience because they are (justifiably) afraid of getting investigated, arrested and prosecuted for practicing pain management with opioid painkillers.

Under-treatment of pain and inappropriate treatment of pain lead to pseudo-addiction. Just imagine patients are being undertreated for diagnoses such as hypertension, diabetes and heart disease. These patients will be subjected to considerable risks with unpredictable morbidity and potential mortality. The healthcare providers in these cases will, more than likely, face medical mal-practice actions. There are pending legal actions filed by suffering pain patients against prescribing physicians and medical organizations for either failure to treat or adequately treat their pain appropriately. As a physician, I inherently abhor medical practice lawsuits, but when there is injustice to patients suffering from chronic, legitimate pain, the patients deserve a day in court.

Pseudo-addiction can be defined as a pattern of drug seeking behavior of patients with chronic pain receiving inadequate pain management that can be mistaken for addiction. Some of the behavioral manifestations include:

- Cravings and aberrant behavior
- Concern about availability of their medications
- Clock watching and day counting
- Unsanctioned dose escalation

A big challenge for treating physicians is being able to differentiate addiction from pseudo-addiction. Chronic pain patients who seek to increase dosages of pain medications in most cases are not addicted, but pseudo-addicted. A doctor who has suspicions should rely on close observation, testing, involvement of other clinicians, if available, such as psychiatrist or drug treatment specialist, communications with family members if trustworthy, and use of medicine agreement.

Pseudo-addiction can cause misery for both patients and their families, just like addiction. It is a sad condition where a patient is experiencing severe pain, but the signs and symptoms are misunderstood and the pain is prejudicially undertreated. Care providers and other healthcare professionals may interpret the patients' request for pain-killers as a form of addiction. Another influencing factor for staff misinterpretation of the signs and symptoms include the pain not matching the diagnosis or because other patients with the same diagnosis manage their pain with the recommended regimen. People seem to forget that response to a painful condition is different in different individuals. If you are given opioids that do not fill enough of the pain receptor sites, you are actually teasing your body. By increasing the dose and filling up all of the receptors, the pain can be better controlled.

Studies consistently show that chronic pain is tragically undertreated in the U.S. and around the world. In June of 2012, an Institute of Medicine report called undertreated pain a " public health crisis " that affects 116 million Americans, and costs the economy about a half-trillion dollars per year in medical bills and lost productivity. The same month, three pain-related articles in the Lancet focusing on post-operative, cancer-related and non-cancer related pain, respectively, found considerable under-treatment in all three areas.

The Journal, Lancet, ran an accompanying editorial pointing to another study by Human Rights Watch showing that the problem is global, and more because of bad policy than because of a supply. In one study of 40 countries, 27 did not consume enough opioid drugs to treat even one percent of patients with terminal cancer or HIV/AIDS. Furthermore, the Lancet editorial added "in 33 of 40 countries, governments had imposed strict, unreasonable restrictions on prescribing morphine, beyond the requirements of United Nations drug conventions to prevent misuse."

So what is going on? How can we be facing an epidemic of overdose deaths supposedly caused by too many prescriptions for painkillers and, at the same time, be facing a public health crisis of undertreated pain? Well, one must take a skeptical look at the numbers the government is touting related to alleged abuse and overdose deaths. In actuality, one will find much extrapolated exaggerations in different aspects in order for the government, including the Center for Disease Control and Prevention (CDC), the Drug Enforcement Administration (DEA), and National Institute of Drug Abuse (NIDA) to throw out a number of statistics in making a case for painkiller abuse.

For example, just one case in point regarding overdose figures provided by the government. In his 2006 Cato Institute paper "Treating Doctors as Drug Dealers: The DEA's War on Prescription Painkillers," Ron Libby explains how determining overdose deaths is often a guessing game. Back in 2001, the DEA concluded that there were 464 "Oxycontin-related" deaths in 2000 and 2001 based on reports from 750 medical examiners across the country. But Mr. Libby points out that "Oxycontin-related" merely means that the drug was present in an apparent overdose death, If the drug was found in the gastrointestinal tract, it was determined to be an "Oxycontin-verified death." Mere mentions of the drug by family members, or its presence at the death scene, were also enough to count the death as Oxycontin-verified. Libby notes that in the deaths in the DEA study, the deceased had also consumed anti-anxiety drugs like valium, 30 percent had taken anti-depressants, and 15 percent had consumed cocaine.

There is also reason to suspect the raw overdose statistics in and of themselves. Dr. Steven Karch, who has written a widely-used textbook on drug abuse and pathology, says because tolerance for opioids can vary so much from person to person, there is no scientific way to definitely say that a death was caused by an opioid overdose. There are plenty of people walking around and carrying on their daily function and living activities with levels of opioids in their bodies that would be declared toxic based on the narrow therapeutic ranges if they were dead on a slab in a medical examiner's office. Karch says, "TOXICOLOGY IS THE LEAST IMPORTANT PART OF MAKING A DIAGNOSIS."

In other words, many of the deaths classified as overdose in recent years may in fact have been caused by something else, but were called overdoses simply because the deceased had what appeared to be an abnormal amount of opioids in his or her system. According to the medical expert, Steven Karch, opioid levels can appear more concentrated after death, and can vary depending on the part of the body from which the sample is taken. It is true that more and more people are receiving prescriptions for opioid painkillers due to the prevalence of chronic pain. That means a higher percentage of people who die today – of any cause – will have opioids in their systems at the time of death. That does not mean that they died of an opioid overdose. Many chronic pain patients suffer from a variety of other ailments and take prescriptions for those other ailments.

In actuality, the estimates of the governmental agencies such as CDC are misleading, and it looks like CDC is getting and relying on the information from medical examiners. The quick and easy conclusions made by the medical examiners or forensic pathologists, as expected, reflected the toxicology results. In my opinion, that our government is using questionable overdose diagnoses in formulating public policy is bad enough, but it is particularly troubling when you consider that some physicians have been charged with manslaughter, even murder, because prosecutors used the same indicators to argue that painkiller prescriptions caused a patient's overdose death. I don't think the government wants to make the distinction between addiction, abuse, and physical dependence.

According to the government's own data, most prescription painkillers are prescribed by primary care and internal medicine doctors and dentists, not pain management specialists. These non-pain specialists prescribe roughly 80% of all prescription painkillers. After more than a decade of aggressive policies targeting doctors with costly investigations and criminal charges, there simply are not many conscientious and well-intention pain specialists left. Many high-profile prosecutions of doctors were successful in sending a chilling message to many practicing physicians, leaving numerous pain patients in the cold suffering. Many of us probably cannot help wondering why our government has been focusing on blaming the prescribing physicians for the drug problem of our society and willing to abandon so many pain patients.

In one of the extreme cases, federal prosecutors compared pain specialist, Dr. Willian Hurwitz to the Taliban. Other over-zealous and over-reaching prosecutors and DEA officials have over the years compared doctors to drug kingpins and dealers, and likened doctors' offices to crack houses. Some doctors were subjected to SWAT raids on their offices, embarrassing them in front of the patients and having all of their assets seized before trial, making it very difficult, if not impossible, for the doctors to put on an adequate defense. Some prosecutors had called press conferences in which they held up big bags of pills the doctors allegedly prescribed, essentially and effectively convicting those doctors in the press. I think, pain doctors and their patients deserve better justice than this!

With fewer and fewer physicians willing to risk their careers and life to treat pain patients in this frightful climate, the compassionate, careful and legitimate pain specialists are likely to be overwhelmed with patients needing pain management, thus, making them prime targets for investigation.

In August of 2004, the DEA posted a set of pain management guidelines on its website. The guidelines were the product of a three-year collaboration between the agency, several healthcare organization and specialists in the pain management community. They were intended to put at ease doctors and patients who worried that the agency's heavy-handedness was casting a chill over pain treatment. Surprisingly, the DEA removed the guidelines from its website three months later and offered no explanation. Some pundits claimed that this was a legal maneuver to prevent the high-profile trial of Dr. William Hurtwitz to use the guidelines in his defense.

As of today, there is still no safe harbor in which legitimate and conscientious pain doctors can operate without worrying about an investigation. What is and isn't criminal will be decided on an ad hoc basis, worse yet, what is criminal versus what is acceptable medical practice will be determined not by other medical professionals, but ny drug cops and federal prosecutors. Under current politico-legal climate, we have already seen unintended secondary effects with pain patients as victims. Some hospitals decided to close clinics for medical pain management. For example, one of the best hospitals in Miami, Florida, with excellent pain doctors, decided that they did not want chronic pain patients who needed to be maintained on medications.

Pseudo-addiction is now recognized as a legitimate and distressing condition and action should be taken to deal with it. However, it is difficult to determine if a pain patient is truly in pain and requires extra medications or is exaggerating his or her symptoms to acquire more painkillers. You can surely look into the patient's background and medical history if available to see if there is any history of addiction. Even then, it can still be difficult to make a determination. This is a thin dividing line between the two, so care and due diligence must be taken to ensure that the patient is not inadequately treated and left in pain rather than risk feeding his or her addiction.

Addiction is a primary, chronic, neurobiologic disease, with genetic, psychosocial, and environmental factors influencing its development and manifestations. Let us look at the true addiction; its symptoms and behaviors include:

- One has to use the drug regularly, and this can be daily or several times a day.
- One tries to make certain that he or she maintains a supply of the drug.
- One will spend any money on the drug even though one cannot afford it.
- One will do things to obtain the drug even though one normally would not do, such as stealing (criminal behavior).
- One feels that he or she needs the drug to deal with the problems.
- One is not afraid to drive or do risky activities when one is under the influence of the drug. In other words, one will continue to use despite harm.
- One will focus more and more time and energy on getting and using the drug in order to get ' high '.

Simply put, an addiction is a psychological obsession about acquiring and using a substance that gives a feeling of euphoria. A person can be addicted to many things. Many people confuse physical dependence with addiction. Addiction is not the same thing as physical dependence, which is when your body is used to having a chemical and stopping it without slowly decreasing the amount you use, will cause adverse reactions by the body.

The relationship between addiction and prescription painkillers is a really complex one, and it is always very difficult to predict. The connection between chronic pain and opioid addiction is a complex interplay between psychological, epidemiological and neurobiological factors. There is no sure way to know who will become addicted to opioids. There may be some obvious clues, such as a previous history of substance abuse, or a family history of substance abuse, or some underlying psychopathology which requires time to discover. People who have gone through traumatic experiences like physical or sexual abuse can have a higher risk for opioid addiction. Mental illness increases the odds too; people with anxiety and depression are more likely to use opioid painkillers on a long-term basis. Nobody should interfere with legitimate treatment of legitimate pain, the question is ' how do doctors or loved ones know whether someone truly needs the pain medications or is misusing them?'

The pain doctors are trying to be caring clinicians and treat their patients suffering from chronic pain with compassion, but also they have to be investigators too; these can be two very difficult roles to reconcile. If physicians and pharmacists just talk more, it possible, I think that can go a long way to help resolve some of the problems and ultimately end in better patient care.

The challenge, for both physicians and pharmacists, of helping pain patients deal with denial and recognize their own addiction is a big, tough one. Patients who suffer from addiction, or who are just on long-term opioid therapy often do not have the insight into the risk that they run. As physicians, you can only do your best, if you want to stay in the field of pain management, hoping not to become a target under the radar.

Chapter Three

The rights of patients with chronic Pain

Incidence of pain, as compared to other major conditions in U.S. :

Condition	Number of people	Source
Chronic pain	100 million	Institute of Medicine
Diabetes	26 million	Am Diabetes Asso.
Coronary heart disease	16.5 million	Am Heart Association
Cancer	12 million	Am Cancer Society

The four most commonly reported pain conditions, according to a National Institute of Health Statistics survey are as follows:

- Low back pain – 27%
- Severe headaches – 15%
- Neck pain – 15%
- Facial pain – 4%

Low back pain is the leading cause of disability in Americans under 45 years old. In 2011, at least 100 million adult Americans have chronic pain conditions, a conservative estimate because it does not include acute pain or children. Not just in the United States, low back pain is also the leading cause of disability worldwide.

Women are more likely to experience pain in the form of low

back pain, migraine, neck pain or facial pain than men. Women are twice as likely to experience migraine or severe headaches or pain in the facial area than men.

Anyway, in the current atmosphere of suspicion, lack of sympathy, political witch-hunting, scapegoating, and disrespect, pain patients have very little medical protection or rights. The sheer mention of chronic pain reminds me of leprosy years past; very few people want to get anywhere near you.

A patient's bill of rights is a list of guarantees for those receiving medical care. It may take the form of a law, or a non-binding declaration. Typically, a patient's bill of right patients guarantees patients information, appropriate and necessary treatment, and autonomy over medical decisions among other rights.

A patient's bill of right was considered by the U.S. Congress in 2001 and failed to pass. Asserting that medical care must be rendered under conditions that are acceptable to both patient and physician, the Association of American Physicians and Surgeons (AAPS) modified and adopted as a patients' bill of right in 1995:

- To seek consultation with the physicians of their choice
- To contract with their physicians on mutually agreeable terms
- To be treated confidentially, with access to their records limited to those involved in their care or designated by the patient
- To use their own resources to purchase the care of their choice
- To refuse medical treatment even if it is recommended by their physicians
- To be informed about their medical conditions, the risks and benefits of treatment and appropriate alternative
- To refuse third-party interference in their medical care, and to be confident that their actions in seeking or declining

medical care will not result in third-party-imposed penalties for patients or physicians
- To receive full disclosure of their insurance plan in plain language.

At least, pain patients have some voices through some organizations such as the National Fibromyalgia and Chronic Pain Association (NFMCPA), I encourage any patients suffering from chronic pain to learn more about it and give it the support whatever you can. Their mission and vision are noble, and their bill of rights for people with chronic pain is fair and reasonable.

Mission statement of NFMCPA:

To unite patients, policy makers, and healthcare, medical and scientific communities to transform lives through visionary support, advocacy, research and education of fibromyalgia and chronic pain illnesses.

Vision statement of NFMCPA:

To end chronic pain conditions from derailing lives by early diagnoses, driving scientific research for a cure, and facilitating research for the 3 A's of treatment for fibromyalgia and chronic pain: Appropriate, Accessible and Affordable.

NFMCPA Bill of Rights for People with Chronic Pain:

- The right to have your report of pain taken seriously and to be treated with dignity and respect by doctors, nurses, pharmacists and other healthcare professionals.
- The right to have your pain thoroughly assessed and promptly treated.

- The right to be informed by your doctor about what may be causing your pain, possible treatments, and the benefits, risks and costs of each.
- The right to participate actively in decisions about how to manage your pain.
- The right to have your pain re-assessed regularly and your treatment adjusted if your pain has not been eased.
- The right to be referred to a pain specialist or other healthcare provider if your pain persists.
- The right to get clear and prompt answers to your questions, take time to make decisions, and refuse particular type of treatment if you choose.

Today state lawmakers across the country are hearing from chronic pain patients who want to reform policy regarding access to pain medications like opioids. In these hearings, nobody denies that the Government has a right and duty to control the illegal use of opioids, and it is agreed that opioids can be an acceptable treatment for patients with chronic pain or intractable pain who have not received relief from any other means or treatment. It is a known collateral that uncontrolled pain can become a mental health issue.

Unfortunately, the proposal of a "Pain Patients' Bill of Rights " comes as national concern grows over opioid abuse, overdose and addiction.

Patients living in chronic pain need a law that protects them. The fear created by what some call an epidemic of prescription opioid painkiller abuse is making it impossible for pain patients to get the medications they need to function with some quality of life. Like many other special groups, pain patients need to continue to fight for their rights, and hopefully with increasing political will power, pain patients will receive assistance which is long-past due. Patients suffering from chronic pain must voice their concern singularly and altogether.

The Joint Commission pain standards say that healthcare institutions must a) assess patients' pain experiences; b) document the results of those assessments; c) provide for treatment of pain, either in the institution or elsewhere; d) re-assess pain after an intervention; and e) teach their professional staff members about how to assess and treat pain.

Chapter Four

Diversion

In this context, diversion may be defined as a medical and legal concept involving the transfer of any legally prescribed controlled substances from the person for whom it is prescribed to another person for any illicit use. The term comes from the " diverting " of the drugs from their original legitimate medical purpose. In some jurisdictions, drug diversion programs are available to first-time offenders of diversion drug law, which " divert " offenders from the criminal justice system to a program of education and rehabilitation. Ironically and unfortunately, members of the medical and nursing professions may also be involved in diverting prescription drugs for recreational purposes, relief of pain or addiction, monetary gain, self-medication for sleep or anxiety, or the alleviation of withdrawal symptoms.

At present, there are four commonly diverted drug classes, and they include:

- Opioids, the prescription painkillers – morphine, hydrocodone, oxycodone and codeine.
- Benzodiazepines, the prescription anxiolytics and sedatives – diazepam, temazepam, clonazepam, and alprazolam.

- Stimulants – including amphetamine, methylphenidate, and modafinil, prescribed to treat ADHD and narcolepsy.
- Sleep aids – including zopidem (Ambien), eszopiclone (Lunesta), prescribed for insomnia.

The anabolic steroids should be included as the fifth class of drug abuse and diversion.

There are different types of drug diversion, including:

- Selling prescription drugs;
- Doctor shopping;
- Drug theft;
- Illegal internet pharmacies;
- Theft of prescription pad forgery; and
- Illegal prescribing.

Pain doctors, besides dealing with opioid for pain, will sometimes prescribe anxiolytics and sleep aids for pain patients with comorbidities of insomnia and anxiety. Nowadays, for physicians with specialized area of practice in medical pain management, they must carry an added role on their shoulders, not that they do not have enough things to do and to concern about in their medical practice. This additional role is being a medical police at all times with their pain patients in order to avoid or minimize diversion. They are expected to be playing the roles of a detective and an investigator while serving as a compassionate care provider. Their colleagues in other areas of medical practice do not have to worry about such heavy responsibilities.

No matter how careful and vigilant a pain doctor is, he or she is not going to ' catch ' every diverter In the busy medical practice. All you need is one diverting patient, which will be enough to get you started with hassles and troubles. Even the famous FBI from the Department of Justice does not solve all of its cases; in fact, there are more cases on its files that are not solved than solved cases. After all, we are not perfect and sometimes, we make unintentional mistakes as human beings. But for some reasons, doctors are expected to be perfect practitioners and be blamed for any non-compliant patients and pseudo-patients. Furthermore, many prescribers are faced with ethical and legal dilemmas stemming from patients who they suspect might be diverting their prescription painkillers. And it is going to be difficult for prescribers to detect this deception because even police officers have difficulty doing so. And if a doctor or prescriber suspects that the patient is diverting or suspects that he or she has a substance abuse problem and the prescriber subsequently deny the patient medications, there is the possibility that this person actually needs the medications and is denied pain relief.

Many physicians, like me, tried to have an honest conversation with the suspicious patients, even though patients do not always tell the truth. Medical records are not always readily available; of course, obtaining patients medical records is made easier and faster with electronic system of health records in 2010s. I had also tried to refer patients with suspicious substance abuse problems to the appropriate facilities with psychologists, psychiatrists and counseling therapists; this was not always possible, and if even the referral was accepted, it would take weeks, if not months for the appointment. In the meantime, patient's pain needed to be taken care of, or the patient would look for other sources for pain relief. This could be dangerous for the patient!

Some physicians deal with diversion by simply refusing to treat any patients with opioid analgesics, but this does harm to patients who need these medications to function better in daily life. Other physicians who are willing to provide care for pain patients run the risk of being deceived by diverters. Diversion and abuse of pain medications is costly to the abusers and to society, and it endangers the treating physicians and the patients in pain.

That is why more and more medical students and medical residents are staying away from the specialty of pain management; perhaps, this is what the government has long schemed and wanted at the expense of one-third of the U.S. population suffering from chronic pain. Has the government solved or reduced the problems of drug abuse and overdoses in our society? The answer is an emphatic "No." We need to understand that people suffering from chronic pain will try hard to find relief from pain at any cost, unless they get tired of living with pain and commit suicide. With all of the restrictions placed upon them and their treating physicians, the patients become very vulnerable targets, and sometimes with tragic ending.

I sincerely respect and praise those compassionate and conscientious doctors who are brave enough to continue providing pain care to their patients. As a pain doctor myself for over 20 years until I fell from grace due to entrapments and collusion in the small town of Sterling, Illinois, I would like to share some of my pain, insight and experience with my readers.

There are many signs of diversion potentially. Although we are supposed to trust our patients and accept what they tell us at face value. It is also important in the arena of opioid pain management to maintain a ' healthy ' degree of skepticism. Diverters come in many forms, so their appearances may be deceptive. It is not surprising that people who work for physicians, friends and even family members may be diverting pain medications. Here are some signs of diversion:

- History of problems with no or hard-to-get medical records.
- Strange stories. Diverters often claim to be traveling through town on business or visiting relatives. One common ploy diverters use is to ask to be seen immediately or to be given a prescription right away with a brief encounter because they have to catch a plane or trying not to be late for an important appointment. They may claim that they have forgotten to pack their medication or their medication was lost or stolen.
- Reluctance to cooperate or tell the truth. Diverters often are unwilling to provide information of any previous providers.

Upon further questioning, they may claim that they cannot remember precisely where they were last treated or that the previous or provider has gone out of business. In many cases, these pseudo-patients leave the office suddenly if things are not going their way.

- History of multiple accidents, minor or major.
- Failure to go for medical testing with different excuses.
- Unusually high (or low) knowledge of medication. Diverters sometimes appear to be extremely well-informed about specific medications. But, they can also appear to be uninformed about opioid painkillers.
- Sing and dance symptoms. Diverters may exaggerate or feign symptoms. Typical complaints include neck and back pain, kidney stones, migraine headaches, toothaches or post-herpetic neuralgia. It was my routine office practice to ask patients for the initial urine drug screen. I discovered one new patient pricking his finger and putting a drop of blood in the urine specimen to corroborate his story of renal colic.
- Insistence on drug of choice. Many diverters are knowledgeable about controlled substances, and they may request certain brands of medication and resist any of your attempt to prescribe generic forms and substitutes. The diverters often claim that they are allergic or that a particular alternative has never worked for pain relief in the past.
- Requests of early refills with plausible stories.
- Use of pain medicines prescribed for others.
- Use of controlled substances from multiple doctors or nurse practitioners or filled at multiple pharmacies as seen on the Prescription Monitoring Programs.
- Loss of prescription or medications with a police report.
- Taking more medicine than directed. In this situation, treating doctor should rule out under-treatment with appropriate actions and investigation.

Honestly, in this modern era of overdose, not just with painkillers, many pain doctors, including myself when I was practicing, are not confident about how to prescribe opioids safely, how to detect abuse, diversion or emerging addiction, or even how to discuss these issues with their patients. Treating physicians can only do their best to minimize drug diversion if they want to practice pain management for their patients, without the protection of safety zone. Here are some suggestions for preventing the diversion of prescription drugs:

- Provide thorough care with a complete medical history, if possible, and careful physical examination. Verify previous provider information if available from patients and document each visit fully, including follow-up visits. Keep in mind that not all doctor shoppers are diverters, some may be real, honest patients trying to find someone to control their pain.

- Use of medication agreements. There are different forms of agreements with various conditions. Very importantly, the agreement should state the reason for which therapy may be discontinued despite possible withdrawal symptoms. The reasons should include any violations of the agreement, evidence of illicit street drug use or abuse or outright diversion. It is crucial that you follow through if violations occur. Not doing so could leave you open to allegations of enabling a drug addict and failing to prescribe controlled substances for therapeutic purposes. I made a mistake of giving some patients a second chance due to their legitimate painful diagnoses.

Medication agreement is not a requirement, and you may not want to use it on all of your patients. It is advisable and particularly important to use one in cases where patients are at a high risk for misusing medications, i.e. those patients with a current or a past history of substance abuse, with comorbid psychological disorders or whose chaotic living arrangements, if known, pose a risk for misuse or theft. Under these circumstances, extra monitoring and perhaps referral to a pain specialist or someone specialized in addiction medicine is recommended.

- Use extreme caution when your patient is using or requesting combination or " layered " drugs for enhanced effects. For example, benzodiazepines and opioid painkillers or anti-psychotics and opioid analgesics.
- Never sign blank prescription in advance.
- Keeping your DEA or license numbers confidential unless disclosure is required.
- No refills for any controlled substances. This was my office policy in my pain management practice.
- For honest, reliable and stable pain patients, I personally want their follow-up every 30 days. For newer, higher-risk patients, they should be seen for follow-up every two weeks.
- Switching to electronic prescribing if available where you are practicing.
- Maintain a dialogue and work with your local pharmacists about your patients. More often than not, it is the pharmacist who first detects a diversion attempt.
- Using the State Prescription Monitoring Programs, if available. At present, these programs in many states are voluntary, and most of them do not provide real-time reporting, thus, creating a missing link or a void as much as fourteen to twenty days in the monitoring process.
- Educating your office staff. Ask your staff to pay attention to what the patients say and how they behave in the waiting area of your office, promptly reporting any suspicions to you.
- Use tamper-resistant prescription pads that expose the word " VOID " when the blanks are copied.
- Ordering urine drug screening on every new patient, even though this is not mandatory or required. This test with

additional cost will provide helpful information for your patient's follow-up visit, if you do not have the preliminary results at the point of care. How often after the initial visit? This depends on state mandates, the individual prescriber, and the patient.

- Writing the quantity and strength of the medications in numerals and letters. This will take a little more time, but it will avoid unauthorized changes.
- Record the name of the medication, the dose strength, the number of pills to be dispensed by the pharmacy, and the dosing frequency in the patient's chart.
- Document and report suspected drug diversion to local law enforcement such as local police, at least it is a start. This will show that you, as the prescriber, are vigilant and careful in your medical practice.
- Checking criminal background before prescribing any narcotic pain medications. This can be very time-consuming, adding more constraints to the already-busy staff and doctors. This practice essentially walks a fine line between the doctor exercising due diligence on one hand and acting as police on the other. I personally did not like it and never did it in my practice. If the doctor chooses to undertake evaluation of patients' criminal backgrounds, that certainly constitutes a best practice, even though it is not a requirement for standard of care.

Serum drug screening. Nowadays, taking good care of your patients is only a small part of your medical practice, especially in the area of pain management with opioids. In addition to the paper work with insurance companies and government payers, and precautionary measures dealing with pain patients and potential drug seekers, time-consuming documentation has become an important part of medical practice in any specialty. In the practice of pain management, some of your patients are probably prescribed dosages of opioids above and beyond the therapeutic ranges but not showing any signs of toxicities or unpleasant/unacceptable side effects. These patients are able to function well in their daily life and productive at work, enjoying their inter-personal relationships. Besides the urinary drug screens as indicated, serum levels of their controlled substances should be obtained to show their optimal stability and hemodynamics. This is critical to avoid allegations of over-prescribing and to prove patients stability and optimal functioning at hyper-therapeutic dosage ranges. If your patient is involved in a motor vehicle accident fatally, you can argue and prove that it is not due to overdose of medications prescribed as many medical examiners would readily and incorrectly certify on the death certificate.

Pharmacogenetic testing. You may want to consider genomic testing to monitor some of your patients response to treatment due to variations in drug metabolism that can result in wide fluctuations in clinical effects. Genomic testing is a new trend in opioid management for pain patients; it can detect genetic predispositions --- such as allelic variation in the CYP2D6 and CYP2C19 genes, which can markedly increase or decrease the metabolism of drugs. Genomic testing can improve diagnostic and prescribing accuracy and can help with patients who are difficult to treat: those for whom no medications work, those who become very sedated with low doses of medication (hypo-metabolizer), and those who are on high doses and are still not getting expected effects with appropriate dosing, the hyper-metabolizer.

Pain catastrophizing

If you practice pain management long enough, you will run into a subgroup of patients, who have legitimate reasons and diagnoses for their pain, subconsciously or consciously catastrophizing their pain. Catastrophizing is a set of negative, cognitive and emotional responses to pain that encompasses factors like feelings of helplessness when in pain. Patients who catastrophize feel that there is nothing they can do about their pain and just can't get the thought of pain out of their heads. They tend to magnify the threat of pain so that it represents more physical danger than it actually does. People who are prone to catastrophizing tend to be those who are at the greatest risk for experiencing chronic pain after an episode of acute pain. They are the folks who tend to get the least benefits from various pain treatments.

The most common tool to assess individual differences in catastrophizing is the 13-item of self-reporting, the Pain Catastrophizing Scale, which can be easily given and quickly filled out in any clinical setting. For patients with a high tendency for catastrophizing, the most common and most proven efficacious treatment is cognitive behavioral therapy with a psychologist or other behavioral healthcare provider.

In closing of this chapter on diversion, I would like to mention narcotic use and diversion among healthcare professionals. According to an article written by Mandy L. Hrobak at the University of North Carolina, Charlotte, narcotic use and diversion among nurses is a growing problem. Substance abuse is the number one reason named by state boards of nursing for disciplinary action.

Addiction is a major driver of drug diversion. Considering the ubiquitous nature of controlled substances in many healthcare facilities, access to these drugs must be tightly managed and monitored. Maintaining the security and preventing diversion of controlled substances is a shared responsibility, NOT just the prescribing doctors.

Chapter Five

History and politics of pain management with opioids.

The medical specialty of treating chronic non-cancer pain with narcotic painkillers is relatively recent, and was started a little more than two decades ago. Back in the late 1980s, doctors trained in treating the pain of terminally ill cancer patients began to recommend that the opioid therapy used on their patients also be used for patients suffering from non-cancer pain. The new therapeutic treatment of pain with opioid proved successful, leading to a huge jump in the sales of prescription pain medications throughout the 1990s.

The potential habit-forming nature of prescription opioid pain medications made some physicians, state medical boards and law enforcement officials wary of their use in treating the pain of non-terminal patients. As a result, many physicians including pain specialists have shied away from opioid treatment, causing millions of Americans to suffer from chronic pain even as therapies were available to treat it.

The problem was exacerbated and sensationalized when the media began reporting that the popular narcotic pain medication, OxyContin, was finding its way to the black market for illicit drugs, resulting in an outbreak of related crimes, overdoses, and deaths. The Drug Enforcement Administration (DEA), as mandated by the Congress and the Department of Justice, responded with an aggressive plan to eradicate the illegal use or diversion of OxyContin and other controlled substances. They are using the tactics and methods from the " War on Drugs " such as undercover investigation, asset forfeiture, and informers. Many of those informers were patients with history of drug abuse or had criminal violations with the government, or disgruntled patients discharged from doctors' practice due to non-compliance and aberrant behaviors. Case in point: four of the six patients in my federal indictments were patients I discharged from my practice after repeated warnings.

The DEA's aggressive strategies have cast a chill over the doctor-patient candid relationship necessary for successful treatment, making the serious problem of untreated and under-treated pain worse, ignoring tens of millions of Americans suffering from the pain. Unfortunately, many people do not realize, or do not want to admit, that the societal costs associated with untreated and under-treated pain are enormous and substantial. Besides the obvious cost of needless suffering, collateral damages include broken marriages, alcoholism, family violence, becoming victims of diversion due to vulnerability, absenteeism and job loss, depression and suicide. Untreated and under-treated pain also cost American businesses hundreds of billions in medical expenses, lost wages, loss of countless workdays, and others. In fact, the pervasive unwillingness to treat patients with severe chronic pain can affect and has affected our national budgets because many suffering patients, after a while, have had no choice but to apply for disability to survive.

In 1997, the American Medical Association states in a news release that millions of Americans continue to suffer from intractable, intense, unrelenting pain not related to cancer due to barriers to pain treatment.

In 1999, the California medical board found, in a formal policy statement, that " systematic under-treatment of chronic pain, which is attribute to low priority of pain management in the health care system, incomplete integration of current knowledge into medical education and clinical practice, lack of knowledge among consumers about pain management, exaggerated fear of opioid side effects and addiction, and fear of legal consequences when controlled substances are used."

A 2004 survey published in the Annals of Health Law found documented widespread under-treatment of pain among the terminally ill cancer patients, nursing home residents, the elderly, and chronic pain patients, as well as in emergency rooms, postoperative units and intensive care units.

Though most physicians approve of opioid therapy for chronic pain, there is still a fear of opiates. Dr. Allan Basbaum from the University of California at San Francisco told the San Francisco Chronicle, "the word morphine scares the hell out of people. To many patients, morphine either means death or addiction."

The word 'drug' has such a bad, terrifying connotation. In our federal legal system here in the U.S., it is such a big net, encompassing seemingly benign marijuana, dangerous street heroin, cocaine and meth, and prescription opioids for pain written by licensed, trained physicians, even though the physicians might have good intention to keep the patients who are suffering from chronic pain and increasingly facing less and less access for health care.

Doctors specializing in pain medicine often find themselves caught in a damned-if-you-do and damned-if-you-don't predicament with some patients. Ironically, some physicians had been sued for under-prescribing in pain treatment, including one California doctor who was successfully sued in 2001 for 1.5 million dollars.

Over the past decade, there were quite a few well-publicized indictments and prosecutions which have frightened many good physicians out of the shrinking field of pain management, leaving fewer and fewer pain doctors in the U.S. who are still willing to risk prosecution and ruin in order to treat patients suffering from severe chronic pain. " The medical ambiguity is being turned into allegations of criminal behavior, " Dr. Russell K. Portenoy told the

Washington Post. He is a pain specialist at Beth Israel Medical Center in New York, and is considered one of the fathers of opioid pain therapy. " We have to draw a line in the sand here, or else the treatment will be lost, and millions of patients will suffer."

Historically, narcotics including heroin were unregulated and widely available in the United States many years ago, and opiates were as readily available for purchase in drug stores and grocery stores as aspirin. The perception changed during the era of the early 20ᵗʰ century when the U.S. government criminalized the common use of opium with the Harrison Narcotics Act of 1914, the first federal law to criminalize the non-medical use of opioids. Furthermore, with the passing of the Drug Abuse Prevention and Control Act (DAPCA) in 1970, physicians can be prosecuted when their prescribing activities fall outside the usual course of professional practice. As you can see, DAPCA has become a powerful weapon in later years as the War on Drugs intensified.

Until the 1990s, the focus of the DEA, as the federal government's chief drug law enforcement agency, was primarily on illegal black market drugs such as heroin, cocaine, crack cocaine, ecstasy and marijuana. In 1999, under much political pressure, the DEA has found a new front for the War on Drugs. In 2001, the DEA had announced a major anti-drug campaign: the OxyContin Action Plan. This shift simply put pain doctors in the DEA's crosshairs as susceptible to investigation as conventional drug dealers. Essentially, the war on drugs moved from the jungles to pharmacies and doctor's offices. In September of 2003, with the 69-count indictment of Dr. William Hurwitz, the U.S. Attorney of Virginia, Mark Lyle, claimed that the doctor was complicit in the deaths pf three patients and compared Dr. Hurwitz to a street-corner crack dealer and his bail should be denied. The OxyContin Action Plan enabled the federal government to prosecute physicians who prescribed an otherwise legal narcotic medication due to unfounded and exaggerated fear sweeping the country. The DEA's efforts linking a legal pain medication like OxyContin to cocaine, heroin, and other prohibited illegal substances was a marked departure from its traditional mission.

In an effort to justify its national campaign against OxyContin, the DEA instructed medical examiners from the National Association of Medical Examiners in 2001 to report " OxyContin-related deaths " for 2000 and 2001. On the basis of those reports, the DEA subsequently announced 464 " OxyContin-related " over those two years. But the conclusions the DEA drew from the data were significantly flawed. Even given the benefits of the doubt, the number was a miniscule compared with the deaths as a result of consumers overdosing on over-the-counter medicines such as ibuprofen, anti-histamine and acetaminophen. In 2000, physicians wrote 7.1 million prescriptions for oxycodone products, 5.8 million of them for OxyContin. According to the DEA's own autopsy data, there were 146 " OxyContin-related " deaths that year, and 318 " OxyContin-related deaths " for 2001, for a total of 464 " OxyContin-related deaths ". That amounts to a risk of just 0.00008 percent, or eight deaths per 100,000 OxyContin prescriptions. By contrast, approximately 16,500 people die each year from gastrointestinal bleeding associated with non-steroidal anti-inflammatory drugs (NSAIDs) like aspirin and ibuprofen. NSAIDs are not as effective as opioids for treating severe chronic pain.

Furthermore, in these so-called " OxyContin-related deaths," many of these overdose victims had other drugs in their bodies. Approximately 40 percent of the autopsy reports of OxyContin-related deaths showed the presence of benzodiazepine drugs; another 40 percent contained a second opiate such as Vicodin, Lortab, or Lorcet, in addition to Oxycodone. Thirty percent showed an anti-depressant such as Prozac, 15 percent showed cocaine, and 14 percent indicated the presence of OTC anti-histamines or cold medications. There was strong evidence that many of the deaths attributed to OxyContin by government officials were not the result of unknowing pain patients who became addicted and overdosed but of habitual drug users who might have used the drug with any number of other substances, any one of which could have contributed to overdose and death.

There is simply no test to accurately determine whether or not OxyContin caused or contributed to those overdose deaths. And even if there was such a test, it was just as likely the drugs came from Internet pharmacies, or friends, or homes or drugstore robberies as from the alleged diverting doctors.

The OxyContin controversy resulted in a fine of $635 million against Purdue Pharma L.P. Rather than dumping the $635 million into a politician's "Look what I Did Pot,". The money could have been directed to a good cause like teaching generalist physicians how to structure their practice to safely prescribe long-acting opioids or promoting patient education about long-acting opioids.

The distinction – which seems especially difficult for law enforcement officials and policy makers – is between physical dependence and addiction. A patient debilitated by pain will naturally become physically dependent on any medication that gives him or her relief; this is very different from addiction. Opioid therapy can give patients the freedom and chance to lead normal lives, whereas addiction ruins lives. At the heart of the debate is the confusion about what constitutes addiction and what is simply physical dependence due to medical needs.

The OxyContin controversy at the time was biased, politically motivated, and media-induced, similar to what the doctors and pain patients are facing now with opioid therapies. The DEA's new mission to thwart the diversion of prescription painkillers was a significant undertaking, resulting in the arrest of 600 individuals from May 2001 to February 2004. Sixty percent of those cases involved doctors and pharmacists.

The DEA's Diversion Control Program is essentially a self-financing, autonomous law enforcement agency that is largely unaccountable to congressional oversight. It is mostly financed by the licenses it require all doctors, manufacturers, pharmacists and wholesalers to purchase, and partly by the assets it seizes when it raids the businesses and personal finances of those same licensees. The DEA's blame and pursuit of physicians for the drug-related problems and the drug's street availability seem arbitrary, unjustified and capricious. Some of them believe and claim that the only way to get prescription pills is to go to the doctors. But that is clearly not the case and being far from the truth.

There were a number of cases in which doctors had had their assets seized even before being charged. This was absolutely outrageous and unjust! Many of these forfeitures result in plea bargains or civil settlements, given that the cases could drag on for years, and assets seizures left the accused with little or no means to live, much less to pay attorneys' fees and court costs. The case of Kentucky physician Dr. Ghassan Haj-Hamed in 2002 is a good example. The DEA in 2002 accused and sued Dr. Haj-Hamed for diversion and distribution of drugs. After more than two years, the doctor agreed to settle with fine and some loss of personal properties.

Pain specialists make an important distinction between patients who depend on opiates to function normally – to get out of bed, tend to household chores, take care of young ones, and hold down jobs – and addicts who take drugs for euphoria, and whose lifestyles deteriorate as a result of using opiates, instead of improving. The DEA makes no such distinction, and by classifying pain patients as addicts, the agency is able to pursue their doctors as "distributors."

Prosecutors also use the threat of imprisonment as a tactic to get pain patients to turn in their doctors, who make better targets. And, of course, once the pain patients can be called and labeled "addicts," the government is free to go after the doctors who treat them as "conspirators" in the illegal drug trade. In the case of Dr. Hurwitz, some of his pain patients were lying and selling the prescription medications on the black market. Ironically, you cannot use this "entrapment" in your defense.

According to the DEA, the prosecution of any given doctor is based on whether there is a legitimate medical purpose for a prescription he has written or whether it is "beyond the bounds of medical practice." But prosecutors concede that there are no specific guidelines or procedures to evaluate either of those standards. The DEA continues to lower its evidentiary standards, making it almost impossible for doctors to determine what is and isn't permitted. The DEA assumes that the Government can investigate merely on suspicion that the law is being violated, or even just because it wants assurance that it is not violated. Essentially, the investigators and prosecutors without medical training in pain management are now in the position of interpreting whether or not a suspected physician's actions are consistent with traditional medical practice worthy of an investigation. It is undeniable that the relationship between a doctor and a patient is crucial for proper assessment and treatment of the patient's conditions. The aggressive and unreasonable investigative procedures of the DEA poison that relationship from both sides.

Investigators often send undercover agents to pose as pain patients, making audio and, when possible, video recordings of everything that transpires, trying to accumulate incriminating evidence against the doctors. I had three undercover agents posing as pain patients in my practice with audio-visual recordings. The A-V recordings did not show any incriminating evidence according to my attorneys; in fact, I told the undercover agents clearly that their request for oxycodone prescription was unwarranted because their pain could be taken care of with hydrocodone, a less potent opioid. One of them actually had taken Ultram and other medications for his pain, while another undercover agent had been treated by her other doctors with Hydrocodone in the form of NORCO for chronic back pain. I denied the request of oxycodone for the third undercover agent and prescribed Vicodin in limited amount to be taken every six to eight hours on an as-needed basis. All of these three pseudo-patients were seen within 30 days for follow-up with a total of nine visits, leading to nine counts in the indictment.

Some years ago before the fervor of the DEA witch-hunt, if law enforcement saw a problem beginning to develop, they would, very early on, go to the doctors or pharmacists and say, "we think there is a problem here." By the same token, physicians and pharmacists felt comfortable calling law enforcement and saying. "Something strange is going on. Come help us out." It was a culture of early consult. Sadly enough, the culture of early consult is gone.

To make the situation worse and harder for the defense of the prescribers, the DEA insists that prosecutors do not have to prove a doctor's malicious intent or desire to profit from narcotic diversion to secure a conviction. The DEA believes that it can bring charges against doctors even if they never actually distributed drugs. For some hard-to-understand reasons, prescribing and distributing are considered the same action when it comes to prosecuting doctors, even though our legal system is very specific on wording. In order to prescribe medications, one must have many years of medical education and clinical training. Pharmacists are the ones who can distribute (meaning dispense) the prescribed drug. Over 90 percent of doctors never keep or dispense controlled substances on premises. I had never done it in my pain practice because it was due to problems of security and liability. In this era of overdose, doctors of any specialty should not keep any controlled substances on premise.

The Reuters news service in the summer of 2012, reported that the DEA used the same tactics of wire taps, undercover operations and informants to prosecute the legitimate supply chains, including wholesalers and pharmacies, and ordered them to follow strict record-keeping and security rules to prevent diversion. The DEA had stepped up its inspections and levied millions of dollars in fines against drug wholesalers for what it claimed were breaches of the rules. In February of 2012, the DEA suspended the license of drug wholesaler Cardinal Health, Inc. to sell opioid analgesics and other controlled substances from its center in Lakeland, Florida, for two years. Shortly afterward, the DEA raided two CVS pharmacies and issued inspection warrants at several Walgreens drugstores and a Walgreens distribution center in Florida.

Many critics said that applying the same strong-arm tactics to the legitimate suppliers as to Colombian drug lords was ineffective and was also causing supply shortages that harmed patients with pain. "Going after a pharmaceutical distributor is not like going after the drug cartel," said Adam Fein of Pembroke Consulting. "I don't believe it is appropriate for the DEA to shrink the supply of prescription drugs, because it has unanticipated effects that have nothing to do with the problem."

Pharmacists were fearful and reluctant to accept new customers requiring prescription analgesics. CVS pharmacies across Florida stopped filling prescriptions written by 22 of the top prescribing physicians. John Burke, president of the nonprofit National Association of Drug Diversion Investigators (NADDI), said that the DEA behaved as though the prescribers, pharmacies and the wholesalers it monitored were the enemy.

The DEA's strategy was also prompting new questions from Congress. Reuters reports that Senators Chuck Grassley of Iowa and Sheldon Whitehouse of Rhode Island asked the GAO (Government Accountability Office) to study whether the DEA's actions are contributing to shortages of medications for pain patients. In his article written in the Wall Street Journal of March 22, 2012, "The DEA's War on Pharmacies and Pain Patients", Scott Gottlieb, former deputy commissioner of the Food and Drug Administration (FDA), publicly criticized the DEA for attacking prescription drug problems in the same way it pursues criminal drug cartels. "The problem is, the DEA may be the wrong enforcer here. It is very difficult to separate appropriate use from illicit use with law-enforcement tools alone."

In the meantime, patients with pain are unable to access a needed supply of prescribed opioid analgesics, are struggling to function. Substitute pain medications often are inadequate and even those are becoming scarce.

Chapter Six

Profiling of a pain doctor

Profiling can be politically sensitive or incorrect today. What is the definition of profiling? It is the act or process of extrapolating information or data about a person or a group based on known traits or tendencies. Or, it is the use of specific characteristics, such as race and age, to make generalizations about a person or group which may be engaged in illegal activities. Criminal profiling is dramatized in the famous TV series, 'Criminal Mind.'

Religious and racial profiling is often looked at as a social taboo for political expediency, but it is practiced in quiet and clandestine ways. The profiling of a pain doctor is very conspicuous and easy, as compared with profiling of a criminal drug dealer. A doctor renders medical care to his or her patients in open daylight, with a known address and posted business hours. Someone from the doctor's office will always answer the telephone calls and make appointments. All the transactions, if you want to call that, including the appointment books, payment receipts, prescription records, and computer entries, can be easily checked and traced. You can find information about the doctor in the phone book, internet and local hospitals. A doctor's office is a safe place to visit without the fear of weaponry. A criminal drug dealer is evasive with everything to hide because he or she operates in secrecy. The criminal drug dealer is hard to find and dangerous to approach because he or she may be armed.

You can be investigated and profiled by the DEA with the following:

- Writing too many prescription painkillers, as compared with other physicians in your community. In fact, you could be the only doctor treating chronic pain patients in the county because other doctors do not practice pain management. Many anesthesiologists that practice pain management are interventionists, doing invasive procedures to give pain relief at the hospital or surgi-center. They typically refer their patients to pain doctors for medical management of pain if the pain is not relieved surgically.

It is a no-brainer that a pain doctor will write more prescription painkillers than other doctors, if his or her area of practice is focused on pain management.

- Complaints of local pharmacists. If one of your local pharmacists is overly concerned about too many narcotic prescriptions by one particular doctor, or if the pharmacist has a personal belief or prejudice against narcotic painkillers (just like some pharmacists refusing to fill prescriptions for birth control pills in the past), the prescribing physician will be in trouble sooner or later, once the pharmacist reports a complaint to law enforcement agencies, either state or federal. The pharmacists take up the additional role of a whistle-blower, and deliberately ignore or simply do not understand the common sense of mathematics. If a physician's focus of practice is pain management. He or she is expected to prescribe painkillers more than any other physicians who are not in pain management.
- Traveling pain patients. I had treated some pain patients who lived about 50 to 60 miles from my office. These patients were genuine and legitimate, crying out for pain relief. They were treated like black sheep in their small

home towns where they could not find any pain doctors. Sometimes, they had difficulty finding local pharmacy willing to fill their prescriptions for opioid painkillers for whatever reasons and excuses. The DEA likened them to the ' prescription tourist ' when there were so many problems caused by pain clinics in Florida, which were inundated by pseudo-patients and drug dealers from states such as Georgia, Tennessee, Kentucky and Virginia a few years ago.

- Cash only practice. Many physicians, usually those in private or solo practice, do not accept insurance of any kind due to the amount of paper work involved in order to receive payments, which can take three to six months. Cash payment is a good way to deal with the cash-flow problems, especially with the rising costs of overhead expenses. Besides, billing insurance for patients with chronic pain was an act of futility in 2000s and 2010s until the Affordable Care Act was passed under the Obama administration, eliminating pre-existing conditions. Nobody seems to care if a general medical doctor asks for cash payments for medical services rendered. However, cash payments to a pain clinic or a pain doctor almost invariably raises a red flag. I guess the mentality never dies: cash only for illegal drugs in the black market.

- Too many patients waiting in the waiting room of a doctor's office. Is there a criterion for measuring the number of square feet for a certain number of patients in the sitting room of A PAIN DOCTOR'S office? If a healthcare provider is good, and able to help patient's problems such as pain relief, how can one expect the waiting room to be empty during office hours? A pain doctor who is compassionate, competent and busy with a full medical practice is often looked at with suspicion and innuendos while other doctors are able to practice their specialties without harassments

- Too many cars in the parking lot. If your practice is in the city with your offices in the high-rises, this should not be a problem. If your office is a free-standing building with convenient parking lot for your patients in semi-rural or suburban towns, you need to watch the number of cars parked in front of or around your office building. If you have too many cars parked, your office can be unfairly and prejudicially labeled as a prescription mill, raising a red flag.

- Patients coming to see you too frequently for pain management. In my pain practice, I routinely gave new patients one week for follow-up for three reasons: firstly, I wanted to see if there were any untoward side effects of the prescriptions; secondly, that gave my office staff ample time to obtain medical records of the new patients, if any. Thirdly, results of the urine drug screen would be available for the follow-up visit. For regular patients on two or three controlled substances including opioid painkillers, I generally prescribed enough for two weeks. For re-visit patients on only one pain medication, they were seen once a month, if they were compliant and medically stable. There was no automatic refill allowed in my practice; all patients for refills of controlled substances must be seen and examined.

The practice of pain management with opioid prescriptions and patients taking controlled substances including painkillers can be risky business; regular office visits with close monitoring is simply prudent, responsible practice, NOT greed like someone would like to label for whatever motives. With the risky nature of the medicines and surroundings, I would not prescribe opioid painkillers for more than one month just to avoid the possibility of accusation that you were not watching and monitoring your patients properly. You can call it 'defensive medicine.'

- Unhappy patients or their family. These could be patients whom you discharged from your practice due to non-compliance and aberrant behaviors, or patients who did not like the limited amount of the prescriptions and costs of the regular office visits because they wanted to get more for their money (this did not necessarily imply that they were drug seeking). Some patients and their family just tried to save money, especially they were on the budgets. As you know, you cannot please everyone; it does not take that many unhappy patients to cooperate with the investigators to cause you trouble and grief. The investigators are not motivated to hear about your rationale and medical judgment about your treatments; they are looking for any information to turn their suspicions into allegations against you, based on fabrications made by a few patients out of spite under inducement and/or threat. One female patient discharged from my practice was so unconscionable lying to the investigators that my wife, who understood and wrote limited English, was writing prescriptions for controlled substances, the office was selling drugs on the second floor and I was trying to trade prescription for sex with her. These ridiculous statements as shown in the investigators reports and transcripts were so false, and no government officials ever considered them perjuries. It is not uncommon for government investigators to ' buy and bribe ' witnesses as one of their legal strategies to make a case against a potential defendant. Worse yet, this patient with multiple painful diagnoses from accidental, work-related and domestic injuries was coached and used by the government to make a victim impact statement for restitution.

Patients who were discharged by doctors who decided to stop providing care for them generally became disgruntled and spiteful; they could be any patients, but the problematic pain patients generally reacted with anger toward the doctors when they did not get what they wanted or demanded. My office building was vandalized a couple of times and my vehicle was once scratched obviously with a key. Of course, the police would never find out who the perpetrators were. It was easy for these few questionable individuals to embark on a 'smear campaign' vindictively against the well-intentioned doctors with vicious rumors.

No recognized standard of pain care exists for prescribing controlled substances, but certainly it is accepted that the prescription of medications to control pain, to reduce anxiety, to assist in sleep or to improve quality of life is often appropriate and medically indicated. Indeed, withholding these drugs when required could well constitute inappropriate care. There are just too many variables in the area of pain management, but unfortunately, pain doctors have become vulnerable and easy targets, and bounties and scapegoats for the law enforcement authorities of this country. Mere hearsays and allegations can subject the doctors to unreasonable scrutiny by people untrained or with little knowledge about opioids and pain management. With further and deeper digging by the curious and mission-guided investigators, many pain doctors will find themselves on the defensive with more and more legal hassles and headaches.

Doctors are not trained to be medical detectives or police in the medical schools. There is just not sufficient time for the curricula. All physicians have the experience of patients not telling them everything or exaggerating their complaints. History and self-reporting is an important part of the H & P; if the patients intend to falsify their medical history for whatever reasons or motives, if is not easy for the well-intentioned doctors to know the truth, especially in the initial visit.

Most of the frivolous cases against pain doctors never saw a day in court for trial; a vast majority of the doctors including myself just did not have the mental strength, the money, the resources and the professional supports to fight against the government which has unlimited resources (money, time and man-power) to prosecute the cases. The doctors, pretty much, were forced to settle with the plea, trying to lessen the pain and stress. Without the moral, emotional and financial supports of their loved ones, many physicians in this boat including myself, might not have survived this kind of turbulence and tempest of their professional journey and life.

Chapter Seven

My long, painful journey

On July 27, 2011, I was served a search warrant issued by the U.S. Federal Court in Rockford, Illinois. Federal and State DEA agents along with the local police departments (the cities of Sterling and DeKalb) raided my two offices. There were at least six agents at each office for about eight hours. I left the Sterling office after I opened the doors for them. They essentially turned everything inside out and upside down. They had to break a couple of the doors on the second floor of my Sterling office in order to get inside the rooms when I could not find the keys at the time. They took away computers and medical charts of patients including anything they deemed pertinent and questionable.

My main office was in Sterling with a population of 15,000, located at a busy intersection of West Third Street and Avenue G. The Sterling police parked a big police truck at the entrance of the property with a huge sign saying ' search warrant in progress '. A photograph of this along with some sensational news were in the front page of the newspaper, Daily Gazette on the following morning.

My full-time receptionist, Carol, who lived about one mile from the Sterling office, met me at the office about 10pm after the raid, we found a big mess left behind including empty cans of soft drink everywhere, left-over pizzas on tables and desks and scattered

Dr. Richard Ng

trashes. Needless to say, we had to do a lot of cleaning up and re-arranging in order to be ready for patients the next morning.

Prior to the suspension of my medical license on October 25, 2011, three undercover DEA agents posed as pseudo-patients with a total of three office visits for each of them. One, a male pseudo-patient, presented with complaints of pain with a history of foot fracture from an injury sustained in a combat and had taken Ultram at above average dose for pain management for some time, and it was detected in the urine drug screen. Another one was a female, presented with complaints of generalized body aches, especially in her low back after house chores; she was treated with NORCO prescribed by other doctors according to the PMP reports. The third one, a gentleman of well-built physique, complained of muscle pain after work-out that prevented him from carrying it on for longer. Two of the undercover agents blatantly requested Oxycodone prescriptions which I refused to prescribe despite repeated requests. I told them that their pain did not require potent painkiller like Oxycodone. Our conversations during the office visits were clearly recorded in their wire-tapping devices. I subsequently, after history and examination, prescribed Hydrocodone in the forms of Vicodin and NORCO for them in limited amount to be taken every six to eight hours as needed. Hydrocodone is a commonly prescribed schedule-3 opioid analgesic by the medical and dental professions and the emergency rooms as a short-term pain reliever. Hydrocodone is short-acting, safe and effective for the treatment of short-term or acute pain when taken as prescribed. To make the drug more difficult to prescribe to the patients and carry heavier punishment, the government is changing Hydrocodone from schedule three to two.

I believed that I did not do anything wrong to those three undercover agents who presented as patients with complaints and practiced within the scope of pain management. As a legal maneuver with the advice of my attorney, I made a plea to one count of prescribing NORCO to one of the three undercover agents without legitimate purposes.

On October 25, 2011, a total of five people including federal and state DEA agents and local police) appeared at my Sterling office and handed me 2-page court documents showing an order for temporary suspension of my medical license. What a fateful day to endure and remember! My staff had to tell the patients in the waiting room to leave and find another doctor to take care of their chronic pain. I went back to one of the examination rooms after receipt of the order, and gave my patient the last prescription I wrote with a brief explanation.

My immediate reaction to this was a feeling of being violated and attacked, but I had to keep my composure and left the office in a very somber mood. I was glad that my wife went to the office with me on that day to help because the part-time office assistant was unable to work. She volunteered to drive home that day, even though I was always the driver when we were both in the car.

October 25, 2011 felt like a Judgement Day in my life. I almost felt incapacitated because I could not think of doing anything else for a living and medicine was my major source of income for about 30 years. In order to reduce unnecessary expenses due to the lack of regular income, I called and emailed three local realtors about listing my office building for sale. Two realtors never responded, and one called me back informing me that his company did not handle commercial properties, even though I had seen commercial listings with his company in local advertisements. I was a licensed real estate broker for many years and was shocked that realtors were not interested in new listings. Here it was my experience of community rejection in a small town!

The two weeks following my license suspension was a very devastating time of my life, mentally, socially, financially and physically. I did not feel like doing anything or seeing anyone; I was depressed and hopeless, and trying to find ways to adjust to the unexpected, drastic changes in my life. A mid-life crisis was an understatement. A good friend of mine suggested that I should file for unemployment benefits. Subconsciously, I had rejected the idea at first, feeling shame and embarrassment. I had never had a chance to be unemployed since the years of high school because I was always busy with school and work. During my four years of undergraduate education at Elmhurst College, I had a full-time job as a machine operator on the second shift, Mondays through Fridays. On the weekends, I worked as a janitor to clean local offices and homes. Anyway, I did receive six to seven months of unemployment benefits.

Finding a job in the healthcare field was practically impossible because the federal indictments are public records. Even though they were charges at the time and not yet convicted, many employers and companies were reluctant to hire me. I was trying to find some jobs as an independent contractor, and decided to give limousine driving a chance. I went to one of the City Colleges of Chicago for limousine drivers classes because a special license was required to become a limousine driver or a taxi driver in the City of Chicago. Driving limousines between the suburbs and the City of Chicago, as a rookie independent contractor, involved a lot of waiting time at the airports, Midway and O'Hare. I was responsible for airport fees, highway tolls and gasoline and car-wash expenses. I was lucky if I earned minimum wages after all of the expenses.

I did not renew my limousine driver's license from the City of Chicago, and worked for Invitation Homes as an independent contractor to do home repairs and improvements with many years of real estate experience as a licensed real estate broker. I worked with sub-contractors including carpenters, plumbers, electricians, dry-wall installers and other laborers. I treated quite a few construction workers during my pain practice and I personally witnessed the physical hard work they did. Many of them sustained injuries to their neck, back and extremities over time, and suffered chronic muscle aches and cramps due to the nature of work. Nobody can perform construction work safely and efficiently while in chronic pain. Many of them need medical pain management so that they can function and work productively, support their family, and achieve quality of life with some dignity. In fact, many of them depend on pain medications to carry on their activities of daily living. Did anyone of them become addicted? The answer is yes with a very small percentage, and it is this very small subgroup that need additional attention. The vast majority of them deserve to live a life they can be proud of, without succumbing to the scourge and misery of chronic pain.

Coincidentally, the Illinois Department of Professional Regulation decided NOT to renew my real estate broker license in the month of April, following suspension of my medical license on October 25, 2011. But the Department kept my license renewal fee. When my brother-in-law, who is an attorney, went with me to the Chicago office of the State of Illinois building to inquire about this, we were told that I could petition for reinstatement of my real estate license with very likely favorable outcome since I did not have any violations of the real estate practice act. I had the real estate brokers license from the state of Illinois for about 25 years without any complaints. With the frame of mind I was in at the time, and the lack of financial resources, I bitterly and sadly decided NOT to pursue any further. Is this injustice or unreasonable power of bureaucracy?

I felt abandoned by the medical profession. The three doctor-friends with whom I had worked professionally and had spent time together socially tried to avoid me. They did not respond to my emails or cell phone calls. I even called them at home leaving voice messages. They were probably afraid to associate with me with the ongoing legal prosecution and ' medical persecution ' by our government, even though they did not practice pain management. One of them was subpoenaed to appear in front of the grand jury to testify about me; of course the prosecutor was hoping for some information which could be used against me. This was his job as an Assistant U.S. Attorney, I understand. At this juncture before the federal indictment, I do not think that the grand jury proceedings, consisted of the general public, probably without medical training or history of suffering from chronic pain, while under the influence of the prosecutors, were able to review the 16,000 pages of information, if ever presented, and to understand the practice of pain management with opioids. My attorney and I reviewed the transcript of my doctor-friend's testimony from the grand jury proceedings and did not find any incriminating information. He was there to tell the truth and facts under oath.

Most of us, including some who had served as jurors in the Grand Jury, do not understand the process. I, for one, had very little knowledge about it until my wife and I received the 89-count indictment on May 15, 2013. I am not an attorney, but I would like to share with my readers briefly about what I had learnt about the Grand Jury process of our country.

A grand injury is a panel of citizens, usually 16 to 23 individuals from the general public, convened by a court to decide whether it is appropriate for the government to indict someone suspected of a crime. The purpose of the grand jury is to protect the fellow humans from prosecutorial abuse. An American institution since the colonial days, the grand jury has long played an important role in criminal law. A grand jury is supposed to act as a shield against ill-conceived, malicious or over-zealous prosecution. Unfortunately, the process has come increasingly under the control of prosecutors, according to many legal scholars and critics. The domination of an ambitious prosecutor has led to passivity that destroys the legitimacy of the grand jury concept; it has declined from a proactive, impartial voice to a passive instrument of the prosecution.

The grand jury served the public in two ways. First, it limited the power of government to prosecute citizens by permitting the grand jury to vote for or against an indictment, and second, it had the power to make a presentment. A presentment was a public report of the grand jury's activity. Through a presentment, the grand jury could make criminal activity known to the public, including criminal conduct committed by government officials, judges, or prosecutors. Constitutionally, it is an independent institution adopted by our founders to protect the individuals from prosecutorial misconduct.

In the early 20th century, a grand jury used their power to investigate and indict the mayor of Minneapolis and force the police chief to resign. Under the leadership of foreman Hovey C. Clarke, the Minneapolis grand jurors paid private detectives out of their own pockets to investigate corrupt officials. When the county prosecutor refused to do his duty, Clarke dismissed him and took over the role of prosecutor. Sadly, much has changed in last 100 years or so.

Most, if not all, grand jurors have little background in law, and they tend to and must rely on the prosecutor to educate them about the applicable law. In actuality, one can often see the prosecutorial leading and suggestion. Not surprisingly, the grand jury tends to follow the prosecutor's advice. When citizens are not aware of their power as grand jurors, they cannot exercise that power to uphold justice. Today, the grand jury is more of a prosecutor's panel, even though it is supposed to be a people's panel.

Furthermore, in federal courts, the jurors may accept hearsay and other unsubstantiated evidence that is normally not admissible at trial.

Grand jury is a strictly clandestine process in secrecy. There is no attorney representing the accused in the proceedings. Thus, they cannot hear any evidence in the accused's favor. Grand juries also face criticism in the area of jury selection, especially with high-profile cases. Criticism focuses of bias and a lack of balance in the selection process.

The grand jury is supposed to be unbiased, meaning that the jurors have no prior familiarity with the facts of the case. Today, this is impossible with the speed and sensationalism of media, the prevalence of digital technology like the Internet, the curiosity of the general public, and sometimes the political tendency of the prosecution.

Federal law provides that a defendant may challenge the array of grand jurors on the ground that the grand jury was not selected, drawn or summoned in accordance with the law, and may challenge an individual juror on the ground that the juror is not legally qualified (Estes v United States, 335 F.2d 609, cert. denied, 379 US 964, 85 S. Ct. 656, 13L. Ed. 2d 559).

Gradually, the executive branch of our government began to limit the power of the grand jury. It became standard practice for the prosecutor to be present in the grand jury room to present evidence personally. Thus, the adversarial roles between the government prosecutor and the grand jury was weakened. Nowadays, the grand jurors tend to bond with the prosecutor and, ultimately grand jury has become a rubber stamp for the prosecutor's indictments. In 1985, former New York Court of Appeals Judge Sol Wachtler, said, "Any prosecutor who wanted to could indict a ham sandwich."

Furthermore, Rule Six of the Federal Rules of Criminal Procedure removed the independent power of the grand jury to publicly accuse government officials of misconduct.

It is not uncommon that ambitious prosecutors attempt to misuse the powers of a non-professional grand jury to harass, trap, intimidate or wear down witnesses that are not favorable for prosecution. Thus, states have provisions in their laws to allow the use of preliminary hearings instead of grand juries, which are adversarial in nature. Unlike a grand jury, a preliminary hearing is usually open to the public and involves attorneys from both sides and a judge.

Grand juries do not need a unanimous decision from all members to indict, all they need is a majority. Like anything else, the grand jury system is not perfect and open to prosecutorial abuse. The state of Hawaii provides grand juries with their own lawyers, trying to sever the close tie between prosecutor and jurors. Such a ' grand-jury counsel ' provides independent legal advice and acts as a buffer between jurors and prosecutors. This, in turn, makes grand jurors more independent and gives their indictments more credibility, and to avoid wrongful indictments which do occur.

Everything was a struggle for me in the period between

October 25, 2011 and May 15, 2013. I just could not find or think of anything that was enjoyable. In the back of my mind, I seemed to be worrying constantly about something worse that might befall me, worse than the day my medical license was suspended. And my fearful intuition did come to pass. In the early morning of May 15, 2013, about 7am, my wife was awaken by the loud banging sound on the front door of our Chicago home. The agents including U.S. Marshall put handcuffs on her after showing her the arrest warrant, which she did not understand due to her limited English language. The female agent, in a distrustful tone, asked my wife where I was. Audrey, being so frightened and shaken, told her that I was in the suburban home of Rock Falls, scheduled to work with some home remodelers that day. The female agent further questioned her if our marriage was in trouble since we were not in the same house, knowing that we had two homes and other real estate assets, according to their exhaustive investigation. I guess that it is one of the tactics our government uses to have spouses working against each other so that the government can achieve what they want.

My wife has been suffering from post-traumatic stress disorder (PTSD) since the day of her arrest. Her awful experience of arrest was further complicated and worsened by the dehumanizing booking process at the Winnebago County Jail, Rockford, Illinois. Someone told her on the day of initial processing at the detention center that she would face deportation, not knowing that she is a U.S. citizen born and raised in Malaysia. Even someone is an illegal alien, he or she has rights and is entitled to due process and not to be convicted without a fair trial.

Fortunately, my wife's terrible stay at the detention center of Winnebago County Jail was short, and she was released the next day with a $2,000 bond. However her painful, life-changing experience is long-lasting, resulting in the condition of PTSD. She gets startled when the door-bell rings unexpectedly. She feels anxious and scared when she sees police car in the rear-view mirror of the car she is driving. She is concerned whenever she has to show her driver's license going through security check at the airport. She does not like to even see security personnel around when she is shopping in the mall. I am very sorry to see her suffering from PTSD, which has been aggravating her medical painful conditions of multiple disc herniations of the cervical and lumbar spine. After all, she is such an honest, compassionate and loving person, and does not deserve the pain and suffering, mentally and physically.

Three agents including U.S. Marshall, DEA, and local police, came to my Rock Falls home early in the morning, arresting me in front of two construction workers after showing me the indictments and arrest warrant. It seemed a very long drive to the Winnebago County Jail in Rockford, Illinois, where I got finger-printed and stripped search. I had to have a buccal swap for DNA sample and surrendered all of my personal belongings including wallet, clothes and underwear. Photographs were taken for public records. When you are being charged with a crime, you essentially give up all of your rights, even though you are read that you have the right to a fair trial. In cases against pain doctors, the trial is never fair, if you have to go through one, because it is a win-win situation for the government with unlimited resources, time and manipulative power. The government does not have to experience any physical or emotional pain, humiliation, isolation, anxiety, fear of uncertainty, loss of friends and sometimes family.

I was held for 48 hours at the detention center of Winnebago County Jail until I was released with a $10,000 bond. I probably had about three hours of sleep while in temporary custody waiting for the bond hearing. There was the almost-constant loud opening and shutting of heavy metal doors of the cells; staff were talking loudly all three shifts, and bright lights were on all day long. Three basic meals were served so that nobody could say they were starved. I saw someone next to my cell refusing to eat most of the meals because he did not like the food and could not wait to eat the food outside.

As their job, the prosecutor tried to make it difficult at the bond hearing, such as demanding unreasonable bail. Prosecution was able to even separate my wife and I, stipulating that we could not see each other without supervision. This plausibly legal maneuver claimed that my wife was a co-defendant and we were not supposed to discuss or talk about the federal charges. This unreasonably and unjustly stripped us of matrimonial privilege and right. My attorney, a public defender, filed a motion in this regard to modify bond conditions a couple of months later, and the pre-trial judge approved my motion to restore our spousal relationship so that Audrey and I could live as husband and wife again. The trip from the Federal court house to DeKalb after the bond hearing on May 17, 2013 was permeated with feelings of bitterness, anger, frustration, sorrow, emotional pain and uncertainty.

The pre-trial period spanned over three years from 2013 to 2017 due to the time my attorney needed for discovery and review of about 16,000 pages of documents from the government. Both my wife and I had to make a 45-mile trip to the six-story federal courthouse building every four to six weeks for continuances and other related hearings. I felt so reluctant and disgusted every time I entered the court building; it reminded me of what my mother told me and my brothers and sisters when we were all living in a small apartment in Hong Kong. " You must try to avoid two places in life: funeral homes and court houses."

My attorney had to file motions several times over the course of the three years to get approval for me to travel out of my geographic restrictions for business purposes. We had to surrender our U.S. passports at the bond hearing due to flight risk as one of the conditions for release awaiting trial. Of course, based on what the government already knows about us with their exhaustive, all-encompassing investigation, they know that we are not going anywhere. All I want is to have this sad and painful chapter closed and out of my life so that I can live again with some purposes, one way or the other and whatever the legal outcome is.

One of my friends jokingly suggested that I should escape to Mexico; this is a terrible and farcical suggestion and I told him not to say it again. Despite the problems facing our country here in the U.S., and the situations I am in with the federal indictments, the U.S. is still the best place to live --- at least this is my personal opinion. There may be other people who will disagree with me.

As we are getting closer and closer to trial, my worry and uncertainty seem to be escalating. Everyone knows that uncertainty is stressful. Every birthday we celebrate with the family, deep within me, I always wonder if the celebration with my loved ones and friends will happen next year. I have the same misgivings for Thanksgiving, Christmas and New Year. I have lost the control of my life and am unable to plan anything, especially for long term in the future. Stress and uncertainty along with inexplicable mixed feelings have caused serious sleep disruption for me. My restless nights have also affected my spouse sleeping next to me.

Once in a while, I used to take 5mg of melatonin and a glass of milk for insomnia before my legal problems started, and it was effective to help me fall and stay asleep. That remedy with melatonin and milk did not work anymore. I started to turn to alcohol, hoping to get some sleep. My father was an alcoholic, and I remember seeing him intoxicated many times at home, causing a lot of unhappiness and commotion. One of my older sisters drank heavily every day until she passed away with lung cancer. One of my younger brothers liked to drink socially and excessively and had to be carried home many times according to his wife. As a physician, I understand what alcohol abuse can do to one's body's and mind, but I seem to have lost control of everything, sometimes, myself. Facing and enduring the several crises of my life (divorce, loss of my medical license, investment losses of my real estate holdings and the federal indictments), I became depressed, feeling helpless. My psychotherapist referred me to the psychiatrist who then prescribed some psychotropic medication for depressive disorder.

Pre-trial services of the court's probation department made home visits regularly; the kind and caring probation officer recognized my depression and alcohol abuse issues. I started therapy with a counselor twice a week and the schedule was later changed to once a week. My wife also received psychotherapy for her PTSD, which is still plaguing her today.

Sometimes, I found myself crying uncontrollably when I think of all of the happenings. In fact, I broke down in front of the probation officer at the Probation Department a couple of times. Is this weakness or expected human emotions? I really don't know, but one thing I realize is that our mind can be a feeble thing. In all of my adult life and before I was indicted by the federal government, I burst into tears three times in my memory. One time was at the Hong Kong International Airport on June 8, 1971, when I was departing for Chicago leaving at least thirty people behind the departure gate, including my mom and dad, other relatives and friends. The second time for my tearful breakdown was when my mother took her last breath in the ICU of Glen Oak Medical Center, Glendale Heights, Illinois. She was hospitalized in her final stage of colon cancer at Glen Oak Medical Center where my sister, Ruth, was the attending nurse and I was the admitting physician. I was grateful for the specialists who had taken care of my mother during her hospital stay.

I found myself crying and sobbing for a long time at my mother's funeral service in church and the burial service at Elm Lawn Cemetery in Elmhurst, Illinois. She left us from this earthly journey about 27 years ago, but I still miss her every day.

One of my younger brothers, Simon, who lives most of his life in England, wanted to visit with me for quite some time. He was able to take a vacation with his wife in September of 2016 to spend some family time with us in the U.S. After all, we had not seen each other for over ten years. My sister, Ruth, and her brother-in-law, Steve, owned a condominium in Naples, Florida, on the beach and invited all of us to spend a week there. The judge was kind enough to approve this family trip, and I was grateful to Steve and Ruth for the air-tickets and wonderful accommodation.

There were so many moments of loud, hearty laughter during the Florida trip, and sometimes we laughed so hard that joyful tears came down all of our faces. We spent some time walking on the beach in Naples, enjoying the sunset over the horizon. We experienced both good and bad days by the Pacific Ocean; on a nice, calm and sunny day, I was enjoying the smooth, peaceful, tranquil movements of the ocean water. We also had a couple of days with stormy weather, with howling, noisy and choppy waves. I suddenly realized with the inspiration that pain in our bodies is likened to the water in the ocean, dynamic in nature, and sometimes unpredictable due to different factors.

My sentencing date was originally set for December 19, 2016, which was changed to February 03, 2017. My two younger brothers arrived in Chicago from England on January 27, 2017, hoping to attend the sentencing on February 03, 2017 while visiting with us for one week. Instead of meeting them at the O'Hare International Airport on January 27, 2017, I found myself in the emergency room at Kishwaukee Hospital very early in the morning due to precipitous lower GI bleeding with chills and profound weakness.

With the abnormal chest x-rays, elevated white blood cell count and other compromised symptoms, I was admitted to the hospital for aggressive treatment. Despite my medical conditions, I was so happy to see my two brothers visiting me in the patient room. I was hospitalized for three nights and four days, and was able to spend three days with them before their departure for England. I was consulted by internist, general surgeon, pulmonologist and infectious disease specialist during my hospital stay.

The sentencing date was rescheduled for February 17, 2017, which was the darkest day of my life. This was a sentencing hearing after the plea agreement, with very little I, as a defendant, could do, according to my public defender. The prosecutor tried to present everything under the sun, including one former patient of mine who submitted a victim statement to the court. I had discharged quite a few patients over the years despite their legitimate painful diagnoses because they were non-compliant with questionable aberrant behaviors. For physicians treating patients suffering from chronic pain, this is not an easy task or decision. This prosecutor presented three people on the stand to make statements, one was a former patient discharged from my care and the other two were family members of patients whom I had treated. Whatever derogatory statements they made, my attorney had no opportunity to correct them. I was told that it was not a trial, but the judge heard all of that whether true or false. It was certainly a disadvantage for the defense.

I was surprised by the fact that the prosecutor was allowed to read the misleading transcript from the Grand jury proceedings of one of my former patients who was a college-educated registered nurse. This nurse suffered several deforming and painful conditions and was maintained on opioids prescribed by other physicians for many years before coming to my care. Without the medications, she would not have been able to function and perform her duties as a nurse. She had written a very considerate, well-informed, supporting letter to me after my medical license was suspended. Her kind letter was submitted to the court with other supporting documents in December of 2011. Her grand jury testimony was given in February of 2012. Her testimonial letter to me and her grand jury testimony were totally opposite and different, and I could not believe the amount of falsehood in the grand jury testimony.

It was essentially a show directed by the prosecutor to impress the judge, while I had no chance to argue or cross-examine. Many of us believe in the American justice, but sadly and tragically, our justice system can be tainted and corrupted by prejudice, political witch-hunting, thirst for blood and spite for a pound of flesh.

The 87-month sentence sent chills down my spine and brought tears to the faces of my loved ones in the U.S. and across the Pacific and Atlantic Oceans.

Chapter Eight

Chronic pain and our veterans

A 2011 Institute of Medicine (IOM) report states that about 100 million American adults suffer from chronic pain at a cost of $635 billion per year. Chronic pain disproportionately affects those who have served or are serving in the military. According to a June 2014 report in JAMA Internal Medicine, an alarmingly high rate of chronic pain, about 44% of the 25 million military veterans in the U.S. after combat deployment, is found, compared to 26% in the general population.

Many service members and veterans with chronic pain also have comorbid conditions such as post-traumatic stress disorder (PTSD) or traumatic brain injury. Many of them are at risk for a lifetime progression of increasing disability, unless the quality and accessibility are improved.

Different people with chronic pain have had different causes, especially stemming from a traumatic event such as war, a physical or sexual assault, a motor vehicle accident, or some types of natural disasters. Under these circumstances, the person may experience both chronic pain and post-traumatic stress disorder. In fact, the person in pain may not even realize the connection between their pain and a traumatic incident. In the military, chronic pain is often caused by injuries sustained while serving or the effect of carrying and lugging heavy equipment for long periods of time. For some military personnel, loads can reach up to 170 pounds.

Approximately 20 to 35% of patients with chronic pain also have PTSD. One study found that over 50 percent of patients with chronic low back pain had the symptoms of PTSD. For people with chronic pain, the pain may actually serve as a reminder of the traumatic event, which will tend to make the PTSD even worse. Survivors of physical, psychological or sexual abuse tend to be more at risk for developing certain types of chronic pain later in their lives.

Chronic pain and veterans is a challenging issue. Between the tough-it-out mentality often prevalent in the military and larger issues like PT SD, pain problems are often ignored. For those brave ones who do speak up about their pain, the road to relief may take years with suspicion apathy and disdain from healthcare personnel, similar to treatments to civilian patients suffering from chronic pain.

While the road to a pain-free life may be long and difficult for some veterans, taking the first step will always be the hardest. There is help, however, in the form of support group and online communities for veterans dealing with chronic pain. These include organizations like Veterans in Pain and Make the Connections.

According to several surveys conducted by Health Services Research and Development of the U.S. Department of Veteran Affairs, many veterans, up to 70% of them, report that pain control is among their top three priorities in their life.

Chronic pain is often wrongly thought of as solely a physical problem, but more and more convincing evidence from research has shown that it can adversely affect your psychological health. One example is depression which is a common side effect of chronic pain due to its persistence.

If you are currently struggling and coping with chronic pain, here are a few tips that can help you to successfully manage your chronic pain:

- Creating a comprehensive pain management plan with your primary care physician, addressing the physical and psychological aspects of chronic pain. The Mayo Clinic recommends the following guidelines to create a comprehensive pain treatment plan:

1. Get a comprehensive medical evaluation (History and Physical). Be prepared to discuss how your pain is affecting your job and life at home.
2. Manage your medications. It may be necessary to reduce your reliance on – and even eliminate some medications as treatment progresses. This is especially true for opioid analgesics which can act as depressants.
3. Try to do regular exercise and enroll in physical therapy. Weight gain, loss of strength, reduced stamina, and limited activity can commonly occur in chronic pain. Physical therapy can be a great solution to these challenges by improving strength, muscle tone and flexibility of the joints.
4. Use stress management techniques. Mental health care, group therapy, lifestyle changes, family counseling, yoga, meditation and biofeedback are all stress management techniques. Consult your doctor to find out which one works for you and incorporate it into your pain management plan.

- Take steps to help you cope and build resilience.

Psychological and emotional well-being are just as important as receiving medical treatment to help alleviate chronic pain. The American Psychological Association offers the following tips to help you cope with the effects of chronic pain as well as help you build resilience:

1. Manage your stress by learning and adopting healthy ways to deal with stress, such as getting enough sleep, eating healthy and regular exercising.

2. Think positively by focusing on the improvements, as little as they may be, that you are making.
3. Become active and engaged by participating in a hobby you enjoy or spending time with friends and family, which will help take your mind off of the pain.
4. Find support by joining a support group and sharing your experience with others who are also coping with chronic pain.
5. Stay socially connected with friends, family members and relatives.
6. Find spiritual comfort.

- Report all the effects of chronic pain to your doctor with the follow-up visits, including any improvements. This will keep your doctor and other healthcare provider up-to-date with your symptoms, worse or better, so he or she can develop an ideal and personalized treatment plan.
- Reaching out for support. Don't be afraid because there are many people in your situations; furthermore, reaching out is a sign of strength. If you notice your pain is having negative impact on the ways you relate to others – family members, children, your spouse or friends – your experience at work or your outlook on life, reach out to one of the following resources:

1. Log onto Real Warriors Live Chat or call 866-966-1020, where you can speak with a trained health resource consultant who is ready to talk, listen and provide the guidance and resources you are looking for.
2. Visit a Vet Center, a community-based center, operated by the Department of Veterans Affairs, that offers counseling and outreach services.
3. Speak to a patient advocate who can help coordinate your care and make the treatment process easier for

you. To speak with a Patient Advocate, contact your regional VA facility.

Taking steps to proactively manage both the physical and psychological effects of your chronic pain will initiate a process of healing and help you ultimately better cope with the potentially devastating effects of chronic pain. All people with chronic pain deserve better treatment, especially our veterans. People suffering from chronic pain are 100 million strong in number, a very large segment of the U.S. population. The veterans with pain, working and banding together with their civilian counterparts can be a strong political voice to decry the tyranny of bureaucratic apathy and prejudice of pain patients, over-reach of power to interfere with legitimate pharmaceutical wholesalers and manufacturers, witch-hunting and persecution of well-intentioned and conscientious prescribers, resulting in unnecessary suffering of many citizens with chronic pain and violation of their constitutional rights to accessible and compassionate health care.

I am glad that there has been more awareness about the high suicide rates among veterans in the past decade, but we can do much more for them and their family. Their suicide rate is about 50% higher than non-military civilians, and this set them apart from veterans of past generations. Men in the military are three times more likely than women to take their own lives.

A recent VA study estimated that an average 22 veterans die by suicide every day in the United States; and there is some evidence that the suicide rate has been rising unabated. This is horrible and astounding! Many brave, patriotic men and women who served our country are living through painful, traumatic experiences during deployment. Chronic pain and post-traumatic stress disorder are some of the reasons veterans may turn to drugs and alcohol as a coping mechanism to deal with the painful, traumatic memories, anxiety, and feelings of depression and hopelessness.

A study conducted by investigators at the University of Michigan in Ann Arbor showed that back pain, migraine, and psychogenic pain were associated with an increased risk for suicide. Although some of the risk appears to be due to co-existing mental health problems, there may be something about the experience of pain that also contributes directly to suicide risk, according to the results of the study. It is undeniable that individuals suffering from chronic pain are at increased risk for suicidal thoughts and behaviors.

According to a large study published online in the journal of JAMA Psychiatry with more than 4.8 million people who received care from the U.S. Veterans Health Administration, individuals enduring chronic back pain or migraine are more likely to attempt suicide, whether or not they also suffer from depression or another psychiatric condition. Back pain is the second most common pain complaint among patients from the Veterans Health Administration, behind only arthritis. Dr. Ritchie, a retired Army colonel and psychiatrist said the study clearly reinforces the link between pain and suicide. She said, " It makes sense that pain is a risk factor for suicide, and it can be the straw that breaks the camel's back in terms of a person's decision not to go on."

Studies conducted by researchers at the National Center for Veterans Studies at the University of Utah in Salt Lake City found other clues as to why suicide rates are high among military personnel and veterans. Members of military services who suffer from traumatic brain injury (TBI), are facing a higher risk of suicide. Traumatic brain injuries can be painful and persistent and they include concussion, cranial fractures, cerebral contusion and traumatic intra-cerebral hemorrhage.

People with pain do not choose to be in pain, just as people with mental disorders such as depression do not choose their illness. Not everyone with chronic pain has a mental disorder or is at risk for suicide. If you are concerned about someone considering suicide, take it seriously. You can get help from the American Foundation for Suicide Prevention or visit the ' Suicide Help ' page on the nonprofit website HelpGuide.org. I hope to help my readers in chronic pain find the support they need to get them through the toughest times.

Post-traumatic stress disorder (PTSD) may alter the way the brain handles pain, according to some recent studies. About half of the veterans in the U.S. have PTSD. A single traumatic experience can set off many different levels of pain, whether emotional or physical. The person in pain may not even realize the connection between their pain and a traumatic event.

Survivors of physical, psychological or sexual abuse tend to be more at risk for developing certain types of chronic pain later in their lives. One study found that 51% of patients with chronic low back pain had PTSD symptoms. Another study found the prevalence of pain among patients with PTSD to fall between 45 – 80%.

A large number of Iraq and Afghanistan veterans have survived their injuries from wars and now face pain and mental health problems, particularly PTSD. According to a VA study published in the Journal of American Medical Association, veterans of those two wars with chronic pain and PTSD were more likely to be prescribed opioid medications for pain management. At the present time, very little is known about the association of mental health disorders and prescription opioid use.

PTSD is a complex condition that cannot be treated solely by drugs. More research is being done to better understand the role of opioid in the management of chronic pain and PTSD. People suffering from PTSD may become either de-sensitized or hyper-sensitized to pain. To combat this, many of them self-medicate their pain through substance abuse. As sensitivity to pain increases, users create an even faster track to addiction when they increase their doses and abuse drugs.

While chronic pain and PTSD are conditions that may often occur together, their relationship to one another is not always obvious and is often overlooked. This is because healthcare providers, family and patients may be focusing on the pain issues. There is such a close relationship between chronic pain and PTSD that they have been quoted as " mutually maintaining conditions ", because the presence of both chronic pain and PTSD can increase the severity of symptoms of either condition.

PTSD is not curable, but it is definitely treatable. Its treatment usually involves a combination of psychotherapy (counseling) and careful medical management. Many PTSD patients have found encouraging and lasting relief, but you must remain vigilant for returning symptoms and future triggers.

Here are the symptoms of PTSD:

- Flashbacks
- Nightmares
- Difficulty falling or staying asleep
- Panic attack
- Depression
- Substance abuse
- Emotional outburst or rage
- Thrill seeking
- Withdrawing from situations that remind the person of traumatic experience
- Suicidal thoughts or action

Chapter Nine

Chronic pain and Complementary Medicine

According to the data from the National Institute of Health's National Center for Complementary and Alternative Medicine (NCCAM), pain is the most common reason Americans turn to complementary and alternative health practices. Josephine P. Briggs, M.D., Director of NCCAM, in her news release for NIH and VA on September 25, 2014, said, " The need for non-drug treatment options is a significant and urgent public health imperative. We believe the research will provide much-needed information that will help our military and their family members, and ultimately anyone suffering from chronic pain and related conditions ".

Almost all of my patients referred to me by physicians for opioid pain management, or came to me by words of mouth from other patients had tried other modalities of pain treatment including surgical and invasive interventions (under local and/or general anesthesia), non-steroidal anti-inflammatory drugs (NSAIDs), tricyclic antidepressants, anticonvulsant medications, muscle relaxants, and some complementary treatment modalities for pain. I would like to talk about some of these alternative treatment modalities and encourage you to give it a try for your pain if you have not already done so.

- Cognitive behavioral therapy (CBT). In a 2010 study, patients who participated in group talk therapy for three months had twice the improvement in chronic low back pain than those who didn't. In a UK study, back pain sufferers who had 90 minutes of group CBT a week for six weeks reported less pain during the treatment with CBT, focusing on solving problems by changing thoughts and behavior. A year later, 59% said their pain was totally cured, compared to just 31% in the group that did not go through the therapy.
- Yoga. According to the research published in the annals of Internal Medicine, taking twelve weeks of yoga classes led to greater improvements in function for adults with chronic pain versus receiving conventional care like medications or physical therapy.
- Meditation. This practice has been proven to reduce chronic pain in several scientific studies. Research from Duke University found that people suffering from chronic pain saw significant reduction in pain and psychological stress after practicing a form of meditation that focuses on releasing anger. According to a study led by Fadel Zeidan, Ph.D. of Wake Forest University School of Medicine, meditation produced a greater reduction in pain than even morphine or other pain-relieving drugs. The incredible thing about regular meditation is that the more you do it, the more it becomes part of you.

Scientific studies with MRI scans showed that meditation works by affecting the brain on multiple levels, but we still do not know 100% how meditation shuts off the primary somatosensory cortex, which is responsible for feeling sensation.

- Pilates. This is a form of exercise and postural therapy. In a 2014 European Journal of Physical rehabilitation Medicine study, researchers found an improvement in pain, disability and psychological health in patients with chronic low back pain practicing Pilates. Similarly, a Medicine and Science in Sport and Exercises study revealed that taking either Pilates or a general exercise class two times a week for six weeks both improved pain and quality of life.

- Therapeutic massage. According to a study published in the Annals of Internal Medicine, chronic low back pain sufferers who got weekly therapeutic massages reported less pain after ten weeks than those who did not participate. Relaxation of muscle tension and improvements of local circulation and joint flexibility contribute to the reduction of pain sensation.

- Acupuncture. This is a form of alternative medicine in which needles, heat, pressure and other treatments are applied to certain places on the skin. It is a key component of traditional Chinese medicine (TCM). Over 3 million Americans visit acupuncturists each year, most of them for the relief of chronic pain. It is now widely accepted among the medical community, and it is pretty popular with patients as well.

This ancient Chinese healing art has come a long way since 1971, when it first caught on in the United States. In 1996, the FDA gave acupuncture its first seal of approval, when it classified acupuncture needles as medical devices. In the 20 years since, study after study indicates that acupuncture can work to relieve pain with variable results in different individuals. Anyway, it should be part of a comprehensive approach to the management of chronic pain, provided you do not have a phobia for needles.

- Osteopathic Manipulative Therapy (OMT). It is a medical specialty practiced by some doctors with a D.O. Degree from schools of osteopathic medicine. One study found that people who underwent OMT for twelve weeks experienced a 30% reduction in their back pain level.

- Electrical stimulation therapy. Electrical nerve stimulation is a procedure that uses an electrical current to treat chronic pain. Peripheral nerve stimulation (PNS) and spinal cord stimulation (SCS) are two types of electrical nerve stimulation. Here, we are talking about the familiar, common and portable TENS (Transcutaneous electrical nerve stimulation) units which are non-invasive, intended to reduce both acute and chronic pain. The unit is usually connected to the skin using two or more electrodes. A typical battery-operated TENS unit is able to modulate pulse width, frequency and intensity, as determined by the patients. While the use of TENS has proved effective for pain control in clinical studies, there is controversy over which conditions the device should be used to treat.

- Ultrasound, a passive physical therapy modality. Ultrasound therapy is a treatment modality used by physical therapist or occupational therapist to treat pain, and to promote tissue healing.. While ultrasound is not effective for all chronic pain conditions, it seems to help reduce pain in osteoarthritis, myofascial pain syndrome, bursitis, sprain and strain, and pain caused by scar tissue.

There are two types of ultrasound: thermal and mechanical. The type of ultrasound therapy you receive depends on your condition. The literature is mixed on the benefits of ultrasound therapy for pain. Much like pain medications, finding the treatment modality that will reduce your pain is often a trial and error process. If you have not had any improvement in your pain after several treatments, ask your therapist or doctor about trying something else.

- Biofeedback. It is a technique that trains people to improve their health by controlling certain bodily processes that normally happen involuntarily, such as heart rate, blood pressure, muscle tension, and skin temperature. Electrodes are placed on your skin, or sensors are held in your hands to measure these involuntary processes and display them on a monitor.

There are three most commonly used types of biofeedback:

1. Electromyography (EMG), which measures muscle tension
2. Thermal biofeedback, which measures skin temperature
3. Neurofeedback or electroencephalography (EEG), which measures brain wave activity.

It seems to be effective for a range of health problems including urinary incontinence, asthma, bedwetting, anxiety, high blood pressure, chronic pain, ADHA, headaches and others. Studies conducted at Duke University School of Medicine Department of Psychiatry and Behavioral Sciences have shown that biofeedback by qualified practitioners are effective to reduce chronic pain associated with the neck and low back, fibromyalgia, migraine, trauma, post-surgical pains and neuropathic conditions.

This modality for pain management involving psychological and psychophysiological aspects of your body may be practiced by nurse practitioners, psychologists, dentists, general physicians and psychiatrists with special training. The Association for Applied Psychology and Biofeedback is a good resource for finding qualified biofeedback practitioners in your area.

• Hypnosis. It is a set of techniques designed to enhance concentration, minimize one's distraction, and heighten responsiveness to suggestions to change one's thoughts, feelings, behavior, or physiological state. It is a procedure that can be used in hypnotizable individuals to facilitate other types of therapies and treatments. According to the review of many controlled clinical studies in 2003 by Dr. Patterson and fellow psychologist Mark Jensen, PhD, they found that hypno-analgesia is associated with reductions in the ratings of pain, in the need for analgesics or sedation, nausea and vomiting, and the length of stay in hospitals.

More and more research has indicated that hypnosis can play an important role in the management of chronic pain. Imaging studies have demonstrated that the effects of hypnotic suggestions on brain activity are real and can target specific aspects of pain. Hypnosis can reduce the intensity and the unpleasantness of pain.

A growing body of scientific research shows that hypnosis works. When hypnosis and hypnotic suggestions are combined with other treatments, those other treatments become more effective. When patients with chronic pain are taught how to use self-hypnosis for pain management and improved sleep, they experience pain relief and better sleep. People who have learnt self-hypnosis can not only experience significant pain relief, but also report a greater sense of overall well-being and control. You can be trained to use hypnosis to deal with your chronic pain, if you are motivated; give it a try and it may change your life!

- Tai Chi. In a 2011 American College of Rheumatology study, patients who completed two 40-minute Tai Chi sessions a week for ten weeks reduced pain intensity 1.3 points on a 0 to 10 scale. The association between Tai Chi and pain management is not new; there has been increasing awareness of this in recent times with renewed interest for the discipline.

This natural therapy for chronic pain (plus its other benefits) has been practiced in China for hundreds of years. Presently, Tai Chi is practiced globally for its therapeutic effects and it is considered as one of the popular health exercises.

For the physical side of health benefits of Tai Chi, it supports or improves balance, coordination, flexibility, muscle strength and stamina. On the mental (and spiritual) side, Tai Chi helps relieve stress, improves body awareness and confidence, and reduce social isolation when done in a group setting.

Some significant and encouraging research shows that tai chi can benefit people with painful conditions such as osteoarthritis, rheumatoid arthritis, chronic headaches, fibromyalgia, and chronic low back pain. However, Tai Chi is not an instant pain therapy. It works steadily and it may be some time before you can see and enjoy the health benefits of Tai Chi.

The ways in which Tai Chi alleviates chronic pain are:

1. Relaxation
2. Gradual control over the pain medications, which may have some unpleasant side effects
3. Gaining confidence
4. A feeling of community and growing social interest
5. Improvements of mental and physical balance
6. Gradual control over anxiety and stress
7. Gradual improvement of flexibility due to reduction of stiffness.

If you are interested in learning more about Tai Chi, you may contact the National Center for Complementary and Alternative Medicine.

- Spinal cord stimulation. Electrical stimulation of the spinal cord and peripheral nerves and receptors can produce substantial analgesia below the stimulated spinal cord segments in some patients with chronic pain. This procedure seems to have good short-term efficacy but long-term efficacy has yet to be determined. Its high cost and invasiveness would likely limit its use.

Non-opioid adjuvant analgesia:

- NSAIDs and acetaminophen. These are widely used and available over the counter. They are usually well-tolerated; users must be aware of their side effects, and informed their physicians of their use. Because they are so common and everywhere over-the-counter, many people died every year from their complications.
- COX-2 inhibitors. They include Celebrex, which work mainly by inhibiting the enzyme cyclo-oxygenase-2 (COX-2), resulting in anti-inflammatory effects with no or much less gastric and renal side effects. They reportedly have fewer drug interactions and have no effect on platelet aggregation or bleeding time commonly found with traditional NSAIDs.
- Muscle relaxants. These can decrease stiffness, pain and discomfort of skeletal muscles caused by strains, sprains or other injuries. They all work on the central nervous system to produce their depressant effects. It is strongly recommended they be used for a short-term basis only. Soma (carisporodol) is a popular muscle relaxant with an active metabolite, meprobamate --- a barbiturate --- that is potentially addictive.
- Psychotropic medications. These drugs have been used in the management of chronic pain because they can modulate

pain experience and to treat symptoms which trigger, exacerbate, or compound the effects of pain --- notably depression, anxiety, sleep disturbance, anger, and other states of excitation. Under the umbrella of psychotropic drugs, they include antidepressants, anti-epileptics, Pregabalin, anxiolytics, amphetamine, and hypnotics/sedatives.

- Lidocaine patches. These are a transdermal method to deliver the local anesthetic for pain relief up to 12 hours.
- Capsaicin. It can be used as a topical ointment against neuropathic pain. It acts by inhibiting substance P formation at the skin.

You need to discuss with your physicians about these options of non-narcotic prescriptions for pain management because appropriate selection of patients is imperative for any medications.

Today it is hard not to mention marijuana (cannabis) when you are talking about management of chronic pain. Marijuana is a controlled substance, officially designated as a schedule-1 drug; however, more and more states are permitting marijuana to help people with chronic pain.

In a 2015 preliminary study of 59 patients with rheumatoid arthritis, about half were given a placebo and the other half were given a cannabis-based medicine called Sativex. The results showed statistically significant improvement in pain on movement, pain at rest, and quality of sleep for patients on Sativex.

A 2014 study looked at patients with Crohn's disease; half were given a placebo, and the other half were given the drug. The study showed a decrease in symptomatology in ten of eleven patients on cannabis, compared to in just four out of ten on the placebo.

A drug called Epidiolex, which contains one of the marijuana components, is waiting for FDA approval for the treatment of some forms of childhood epilepsy.

Pharmacologically, the principal psychoactive constituent of cannabis is tetrahydrocannabinol (THC). Aside from a subjective change in perception and mood, the most common short-term physical and neurological effects include increased appetite and consumption of food, lowered blood pressure and increased heart rate. According to National Institute on Drug Abuse, inhaling marijuana cam raise the heart rate by 20 to 50 beats per minute and this can last up to three hours.

According to a 2006 United Kingdom government report, using cannabis is less dangerous than tobacco, prescription drugs and alcohol in social harms, physical harm and addiction. Marijuana is rarely the only drug involved in an overdose death. Dr. Lester Grinspoon, a professor emeritus of Psychiatry at Harvard Medical School and author of " Marijuana, the Forbidden Medicine " says that one day cannabis " will be seen as a wonder drug, as was penicillin in the 1940s. Like penicillin, herbal marijuana is remarkably nontoxic."

The medical use of cannabis has several well-documented beneficial effects. Among these are: lessening of nausea and vomiting, stimulation of hunger in chemotherapy and AIDS patients, lowered intraocular eye pressure in glaucoma patients, as well as general analgesic effects as pain reliever.

Here are some of the caveats for marijuana users:

- It can impair short-term memory.
- It can affect your concentration.
- In some people, it can increase the risk of depression.
- It may distort your sense of time.
- Marijuana influences activity in the cerebellum and basal ganglia, two brain areas that help regulate balance, coordination, reaction time and posture. Thus, it can impair psychomotor coordination and throw your balance off.

As of April of 2011, medical marijuana is legal in Washington, D.C. On December 06, 2012, the state of Washington legalized marijuana, closely followed by the state of Colorado. Thereafter, a few other states in the U.S. also legalized marijuana, with the list of states for medical cannabis expected to get longer. According to the official report from the state of California, over 40 percent of Californians who take the drug for medicinal purposes use it for chronic pain. In fact, more and more states are permitting marijuana to help people living with chronic pain. There is a growing body of evidence that supports the use of THC for pain management, especially diabetic neuropathic pain. However, smoking of herbal THC remains a concern due to contaminants.

The federal government recently announced that it will not prosecute users or producers of medical marijuana in states that allow it for medical use. This case, with the controlled substance of marijuana, is truly an irony and dilemma as far as government policies are concerned. Although some experts are not willing to believe it, a growing list of studies have found a reduction in severity and discomfort resulting from the use of medical marijuana for pain relief and management.

According to a few recent scientific studies, permitting legal access to marijuana is consistently associated with lower rates of opioid use, abuse and mortality. One of them, published in the Journal of American Medical Association Internal Medicine found that states with medical cannabis laws had a 24.8 percent lower mean annual opioid overdose mortality rate compared with states without medical cannabis laws. Investigators at the RAND Corporation reported similar results.

A 2016 survey by Castlight Health showed that adults are more than twice as likely to engage in doctor shopping for opioids in states without marijuana access as compared to states that allow it.

Investigators of another 2016 study, published in The International Journal of Drug Policy, reported that patients' use of prescription opioids, benzodiazepine, and anti-depressants fell significantly when they had legal access to THC. Studies of chronic pain patients have found that the analgesic properties of marijuana are sufficiently effective to motivate patients to decrease their opioid use; and in some cases, patients were able to give up the opioid prescriptions all together. A clinical trial, conducted in 2016 in Israel reported a 44 percent in opioid use among pain patients who had access to legal marijuana.

There are more and more evidences that do not support the opponents claim that marijuana acts as a ' gateway ' to the use and eventual abuse of other illicit substances.

Chapter Ten

Pain and Cultures

We know that pain is personal and private, but it is also cultural and a complex phenomenon. The feeling and expression of pain can vary in different cultures. The Americans, in general, have no hesitation or difficulty in expressing and telling their pain. Cultural diversity has a significant impact on the experience of pain, and the need for our regulatory authorities and healthcare providers to acknowledge and understand this is imperative.

Cultural beliefs, specifically about pain, among different nationalities and ethnic groups can affect pain perception and its treatment. Pain, regardless of culture, can have detrimental influences on the body and mind if not properly managed, albeit acute or chronic. Some cultures tend to discourage the expression of pain, implying weakness and cowardliness with any complaints of pain. Some cultures may use the tolerance of pain and suffering to publicize certain ideology and political and religious protests. An example of this is burning of one's body by the Tibetan monks in Tibet, China. Some cultures will show special power and strength with their extreme tolerance of pain, such as standing and walking on burning piles of charcoal or branches.

The United States is a nation of immigrants, and minority populations are on the rise with different ethnicity and cultural background. As the U.S. population increases in diversity, the need for healthcare workers and professionals to learn, acknowledge and understand cultural beliefs, values and attitudes toward one's health is essential to providing satisfactory medical care.

A great deal can be learned about different cultures that exist throughout the world. The experience of pain is personal, and can be undoubtedly influenced by one's cultural identity. Over the long course of human existence, a variety of beliefs evolved about the causes of pain. Humans have been dealing with pain for thousands of years, and you may wonder why there is such an interest and awareness in it now. According to many studies in recent years, it has come to light that pain is not being managed or treated effectively and fairly, and many patients with chronic pain are suffering unnecessarily with prejudice and misunderstanding. Pain is a complex health issue with profound consequences and it must be addressed in order to provide appropriate medical care.

Unrelieved and undertreated pain can lead to serious and even deadly complications for the suffering patients. Nobody wants to relive the pain over and over again without relief. Providing optimal relief for pain allows the sufferers to move on with activities of daily living and become an active member of society.

Our healthcare systems and institutions should teach medical, dental, pharmacy, nursing students and other healthcare workers to understand the dynamics of pain and to support appropriate pain treatment for every patient when medically necessary and indicated. In so doing, it will facilitate a respectable and compassionate bond between the patients and the healthcare providers. It is also important that pain patients learn to try complementary and alternative methods for pain relief such as meditation, yoga, hydro-therapy, touch therapies like massages, cognitive behavioral therapy and others, if available.

In the management of pain for patients with different culture, language barriers can be problematic. This issue may limit patient's ability to effectively communicate with healthcare professionals and can lead to knowledge deficit and poor outcome. Even if an interpreter is available, it may not completely and effectively convey the perception and suffering of pain by the patients.

The culture of patients can be a barrier to providing adequate pain management. This is an area which should receive more attention in order to gain further knowledge and understanding. As the American society becomes more diverse, it is essential that healthcare providers and our government strive to become familiar with different cultures among us in the delivery of medical care. To begin to understand another culture, one needs to reflect upon one's personal cultural beliefs and values in order to have an unbiased relationship with the patients. It would be naïve for anyone to think that healthcare providers are capable of completely removing all prejudices when caring for a patient, especially one with a different culture. One prime example of a prejudice or misconception is that ' pain is a normal part of aging within the elderly population '. This is so horrible! Would you like to have your pain ignored when you get older?

If the healthcare providers and our government are not willing, or are unable to reflect on their thinking and remove their misconceptions, it may lead to cultural imposition of one's belief and value system. This is crucial for our society to avoid because they are in a position of power and can easily persuade others. The desire to learn from other cultures with an open mind allows one to gain different viewpoints as well as shared beliefs and values.

I will discuss certain selected ethnic groups based on their response to pain and their beliefs of the origin of pain. These cultures are chosen because their populations, namely, the Hispanic Mexicans and the Asian Chinese, have been increasing rapidly and exponentially. However, one must be careful not to generalize or pigeonhole someone from a specific culture.

As Camphina-Bacote stated, "It is crucial to remember that no individual is a stereotype of one's culture of origin but rather a unique accumulation of life experiences of the process of acculturation to other cultures.

About 34 million Hispanics of Mexican origin resided in the U.S. in 2012, according to the Census Bureau. Mexicans are by far the biggedt ethnic group, accounting for two thirds of the U.S. Hispanic population in 2012. The state with the largest percentage of Hispanics and Latinos is New Mexico at about 47% as of 2012. According to California demographic statistics, Hispanics and Latinos were the largest single racial/ethnic group in the state in 2014, making up 39% of California's population. This makes California the second state, behind New Mexico, where whites are not the majority.

The vast majority of the Mexican Americans ascribe to Roman Catholic rituals and beliefs. They tend to believe the role of God in one's health and illness. Illness and pain may be seen as a discord between elements or as a punishment from God. One of the beliefs is that someone with evil power or thoughts can cause one to get sick or have pain simply by giving the person the ' evil eye '. One way in which to remove the ' evil eye ' is to seek folk healers. It is thought that the person who creates the ' evil eye ' must touch the sick, suffering person to dispel or remove the illness.

Family is a vital part of the Mexican culture and often plays a role in healthcare seeking behavior. The mother is deemed the head of the household, and thus the matriarch becomes the decision-maker of when one is to seek medical intervention. Experience of pain in the Mexican culture may be expressed as emotional self-restraint and stoic inhibition of strong feelings. Machismo is a view that is often held by Mexican men. Being tough can lead to serious consequences especially if the person is in need of medical intervention. To assist in dealing with machismo, one should let the patients know that despite their need for medical help, they are still considered to be strong and courageous.

Although machismo prevails in Mexican society, it can be set aside when facing severe, unrelenting pain. One must be aware that, due to religious belief, some patients may not want to have pain relief because it is an act of God and therefore the pain should be endured. It is important that healthcare providers educate the patients on the need for controlling pain and the possible consequences that can occur if the pain is not properly treated.

Misconceptions and misinformation about pain must be dispelled and clarified to reduce human suffering!

According to USA Today in 2014, the U.S. population growth was tilting toward Asians. For the second straight year, net immigration by Asians topped that of Hispanics, the Census Bureau reported. Asian Americans include Chinese (including Taiwanese), Filipinos, Indians, Vietnamese, Koreans, Japanese, Cambodians and a few others.

From 2000 to 2010, the Asian and Asian American population grew faster than any other ethnic groups, increasing by 46%. The trend is continuing, according to official estimates, and Asian Americans, at the present level, comprise about 6% of the entire U.S. population. The state of California has the largest Asian-American population at about 8.1 million in 2014.

In the Chinese culture, showing emotion such as pain may be seen as a sign of weakness in one's character. Many Chinese patients may suffer quietly, so healthcare providers need to look for non-verbal cues of pain. Education is highly valued within the culture and therefore it is important that patients be provided with valid and reliable information. As a traditional culture for thousands of years under imperial rule, those in respected or powerful positions such as doctors are rarely challenged even if the patients do not agree with the medical regimen being followed. For them, it is just inappropriate to challenge those in authoritative roles. In Chinese society and families, pain is often suppressed and internalized. The person is afraid to express his or her pain, even if he or she tries to express the feeling of pain, it is usually ignored or minimized.

It is not uncommon that patients with pain often run into resistance from parents, their spouses and grown-up children. These family members, not only less than sympathetic, often criticize the patients (supposedly their loved ones) for attention-seeking, exaggerating the pain and wasting money and time. These situations can also be seen in our American society. I had known some of my patients who had to borrow money from friends in order to be able to see me because their spouses and parents refused to help them financially.

In China, opioid use and opioid prescriptions are less common due to cultural differences in pain perception and management. In the Chinese culture, pain itself is not generally considered a disease that requires immediate attention and treatment. One is expected to try to tough it out. We will look at management of post-operative pain in China. In China, patients are usually bed-bound for some time after surgeries, especially the major ones, and taken care of by family members. According to tradition, a woman is to stay in bed at home for one month after giving birth; grandparents and other close family members usually volunteer fervently to care for the newborn and the mother who just went through labor and delivery. In situations like this with plenty of rest, assistance and social interactions, there is less need for powerful painkillers. On the other hand, American post-op patients, in this case, post-partum, pride themselves as independent and request a quick return to normal life. This usually cannot be done without pain medications that provide quick pain relief, even for a short term.

The traditional philosophy and idea of balance or harmony exists within the belief of: yin and yang. The yin and yang are essentially opposites of each other that keeps one another in balance. Illness including pain is often seen as a personal burden when a family member becomes sick. The older generation like the parents will not let their children (adults) know of any discomfort or pain, trying to hide it from the rest of the family until their symptoms become too obvious to cover up. One sad example is my own mother, who had rectal bleed for quite some time while I was receiving my medical education. Her chronic blood loss was kept as a secret until she became so weak that we had to admit her to the hospital. Her final diagnosis was cancer of colon and she survived five years after that. We know that colon cancer is preventable with screening and early diagnosis. To tell you the truth, I am still living with the guilt for not having discovered her problems early.

It is not uncommon for many Chinese patients who are ill

to seek ' traditional methods ' of healing such as moxibustion or cupping, acupuncture, and herbal supplements or prescriptions from the TCM practitioners. The cultural notion that pain is inevitable in life and the medications will not provide adequate relief is also a common belief. Some may consider masking the pain with analgesics, either prescription or over-the-counter, can disturb the natural course of yin and yang.

Chapter Eleven

Chronic Pain and Nutrition

Chronic pain without a visible and obvious cause is one of the most difficult health problems to manage, because many people often assume that you are just making it up for attention (especially if you look healthy otherwise, as if anyone could tell how healthy someone is by looking at them!). Doctors are reluctant to prescribe strong painkillers for patients who complain about pain but do not have any outer sign to show for it. The tendency for doctors NOT to prescribe painkillers seems to be getting worse under the strong arms of the DEA and the fear of investigation by the government.

But if you are like the vast majority of people suffering from chronic pain, you are definitely not making it up, and it does not have to have a visible and obvious cause to be ' legitimate ' pain. While waiting for the political winds to change course, you need to look for other alternatives to help with your pain, if you have not already done so. In this chapter, we are going to look at the nutritional aspect of pain management.

No diet can magically get rid of your chronic pain; obviously, if you have chronic pain secondary to a disease process, the first step is to go to your physician for that disease. No single food can completely stop chronic pain, but a healthy diet is a powerful part of your pain management strategy. There is no magic pill, including prescription painkillers, that will make the pain go away, but considering what diet can do for your pain sounds like a good idea. You will have nothing to lose anyway, with a healthful diet, except for the pain.

For example, the Mediterranean diet is rich in fruits and vegetables, whole grains and unsaturated fats. These foods can help build strong bones and muscles, and --- in some cases --- can even fight pain. A wholesome diet also helps prevent pain-aggravating weight gain and boosts your energy levels and mood so you can cope more effectively and comfortably. If you suffer from other medical conditions in addition to your pain, a healthy diet is even more important.

Many people turn to the so-called comfort foods when in pain or under stress. Well, it is not so bad as long as you eat it in moderation with portion control. The problems arise, however, when you over-indulge in it. Let us start with what you should not eat if you have chronic pain. Today, with 70%of the U.S. population are overweight and obese, most Americans consume more calories than they actually need. Many of the foods they choose are also high in saturated fats, refined sugar and salt. Such diets, besides making you prone to obesity, may actually increase the intensity of your chronic pain.

Such diets also increase inflammation in your body, which can be of particular concern if you have sore muscles or joint pain.

EXCESS WEIGHT, EXTRA PAIN!

Researchers have found that people with chronic pain who are also overweight and obese tend to report more severe pain levels than those who maintain a healthy weight. For patients with chronic pain in the spine, hips, knees and feet, excess weight can aggravate the pain.

Nutritional approaches to pain management can involve both changes in diet and the use of dietary supplements including vitamins, minerals, enzymes and other substances. The strategy can be used to prevent pain such as migraine headaches, or promote the relief of pain, or reduce inflammation.

With the topic of inflammation getting more and more medical attention and public interest these days due to its many positive roles in diseases, it is only natural that more and more people are looking into the so-called anti-inflammatory diet. Inflammation, sometimes, is a good thing --- it protects the body when there is injury --- but it can also be painful. Since inflammation and the immune system are closely intertwined, an anti-inflammatory diet should be a healthy, balanced diet with a focus on certain foods that also have beneficial anti-inflammatory properties. However, if you have certain medical conditions in which inflammation may have a questionable role, you should inform and work with your physician while adopting the diet. Please be informed that an anti-inflammatory diet takes some time to work, and your patience and fortitude is necessary.

Chronic inflammation in your body can both trigger the nociceptors to feel pain and make them more sensitive to other stimuli. Inflammation is linked with chronic pain whether the pain comes from another disease (e.g. cancer), whether it comes from mechanical stress (e.g. poor posture, abnormal bone structure, back pain from sitting all day), or whether it does not have any identifiable cause at all.

With certain inflammatory conditions, or autoimmune disease such as --- rheumatoid arthritis, osteoarthritis, fibromyalgia, celiac disease, Crohn's disease (inflammatory bowel disease), and multiple sclerosis --- the immune system's response is inflammatory, even when there is no threat. Avoidance of inflammatory foods as listed below can help reduce and soothe the inflammatory response, thus, alleviating the symptoms.

- Cow milk. About 60% of the world's population suffers from cow milk intolerance or milk allergy, which is an allergy to casein (or milk protein). Cow milk is very inflammatory, causing a host of health problems including upset stomach, diarrhea, constipation, hives and breathing trouble.

- Fatty red meat. These include ribs, ground beef, burgers, and fatty cuts of steaks; they are inflammatory due to the high content of animal fats. These bad trans, saturated and hydrogenated fats have been linked to some health problems such as diabetes, cardiovascular disease and cancer in many medical studies.

- Cheese. It is inflammatory, particularly of the high-sodium, processed variety. A 2013 Harvard study backs up this claim, finding that cream cheese rapidly alters the micro-organisms residing in the intestinal tract, leading to high levels of inflammation in the gut.

- Margarine. It contains high levels of saturated fat and trans-fatty acids, known to exacerbate the inflammatory response in the body. It is best to avoid margarine and use olive oil instead.

- Alcohol. According to many studies including those at Harvard Medical School, excessive alcohol consumption is linked to chronic inflammation, especially in the liver, leading to cancerous tumor growth over time.

- Cured, processed meats. They contain a combination of salt, nitrite, nitrates or sugar, and are known inflammatory offenders that have been linked to autoimmune conditions. These meats include hot dogs, sausages, bologna, and other lunch meats.

- Food additives. Monosodium Glutamate (MSG) is found in many processed foods. MSG acts as an excitatory neurotransmitter that may stimulate pain receptors. Aspartame, an artificial sweetener found in some diet sodas and many sugar-free beverages, is part of a chemical group called excitotoxins, which activate neurons that can increase sensitivity to pain. According to studies from the Center for Asthma and respiratory Diseases at the University of Newcastle in Australia, MSG and aspartame have been linked to aggravating inflammatory symptoms in those with chronic asthma.

Most people do not see the relationship between what they eat and their chronic pain. Here are some basic guidelines for healthy eating:

- Eating more fruits and vegetables.
- Eating more beans and whole grains.
- Cutting out refined, processed foods.
- Drinking more water. If you can't stomach plain water, try adding lemon or orange slices.

Let us look at some of the anti-inflammatory foods that may reduce your experience of pain and promote a sense of well-being:

- Tart cherries. According to studies in 2012 by researchers from Oregon Health and Science University, they have the highest anti-inflammatory content of any food. Research has found that they can help treat gout, a painful form of arthritis that causes swollen, hot, red joints caused by a buildup of uric acid in the blood. Other studies noted that athletes, who drank tart cherry juice for seven days prior to an intense running event, showed much less muscle pain after the race.
- Berries. These include strawberries and blueberries. Studies have shown that regular consumption of these fruits reduce the levels of CRP, an inflammation marker, in the blood. They have powerful anti-inflammatory properties in addition to their many other nutrients.
- Olive oil. Take a cue from the healthy Mediterranean cuisines and make extra-virgin olive oil a staple in your dressings and sauces. Swap the butter with saturated fats with healthier choices like olive oil. It contains a compound, oleocanthal, which has been shown to have a similar effect

as non-steroidal anti-inflammatory drugs (NSAIDs) such as ibuprofen as painkillers. It can ease your inflamed joints and lessen your morning stiffness, according to some nutritional studies.

- Garlic and onion. These pungent vegetables are known boosters for the immune system. Studies have shown that they work similarly to NSAID painkiller in our body like ibuprofen.

- Ginger and turmeric. These spices are common in Asian and Indian cooking, with strong anti-inflammatory properties. Their antioxidants are boosters for the immune system. Ginger is a wonder root; it can combat nausea and motion sickness, and fight off pain with its anti-inflammatory properties. One study showed that ginger, specifically in the form of a 250mg or 500mg capsule of powdered ginger, was as effective as ibuprofen in relieving menstrual cramp and pain.

Turmeric is one of the most powerful known anti-inflammatory herbs, helping you fight arthritis, gout, autoimmune disease, sciatic, and other inflammatory conditions.

- Beets. The red vegetable has high content of antioxidants which have been shown to reduce inflammation, in addition to its many other nutrients for good health.

- Tomatoes. They are rich in lycopene, which has strong anti-inflammatory properties. In a recent study from Illinois Institute of Technology (IIT), subjects ate one meal containing tomatoes and one meal that did not have tomatoes. They were tested for a marker of inflammation after both meals; their inflammation levels were found to be significantly lower after the tomato meal.

- Peppers. Colorful vegetables like red peppers should be a part of a healthy diet. Hot peppers like chili and cayenne are rich in capsaicin, a chemical that is used in topical cream to reduce pain and inflammation.

- Black peppers. Piperine is a powerful compound in black peppers; black peppers have been used for centuries in Eastern Medicine to treat multiple health conditions including inflammation. Recent animal studies have shown that piperine may have the ability, not only to decrease inflammation, but also the ability to interfere with the formation of new fat cells, a reaction known as adidogenesis, resulting in a decrease in body fat, waist size and cholesterol levels.

- Soy. Several scientific studies have suggested that, isoflavones, compounds found in soy products may help lower CRP and inflammation levels in the body. Participants with knee pain reported less discomfort and used fewer pain medications after eating soy protein every day for three months, according to Oklahoma State University.

- Nuts. They include cashew, walnuts and almonds; they contain heart-healthy fats which can also help fight inflammation along with their packed antioxidants.

- Dark leafy greens. The vitamin E in these vegetables such as kale, spinach and broccoli may play a key role in protecting the body from the pro-inflammatory molecules called cytokines. They are also rich in phytochemicals called glucosinolates, which are powerful antioxidants.

- Whole grains. The high fiber content in brown rice, oats and quinoa has been shown to reduce levels of CRP, a marker of inflammation, in the body, ideal for people suffering from joint pain.

- Fatty fish. They include salmon, tuna, mackerel and sardines which are rich in omega-3 fatty acids. These healthy fats have been shown to lower inflammation with decreased levels of CRP. Omega-3 fatty acids have been shown to reduce arthritic pain, especially in the neck and back. In one study, the relief of pain experienced from consuming omega-3 fatty acids in the form of a fish oil supplement was comparable to the relief experienced from taking ibuprofen. So, start having some fish dishes two to three times a week (not the fried version) and enjoy your life with less pain.

One large scale, prospective study of women ages 55 to 89 in Sweden showed a 29% decreased risk of developing rheumatoid arthritis among participants who ate two or more servings of fish per week compared to women who ate one serving or less per week.

Fish is also high in vitamin D, the bone-building nutrient. Bone loss can often occur around inflamed joints, and steroid injections and medications can be harsh on your bones. There is a strong link between low levels of vitamin D and chronic pain. Recent studies have shown that a diet rich in vitamin D may help ease chronic pain. A 2009 study found that patients deficient in vitamin D required almost twice as much pain medication as patients with adequate levels. Supplementing with vitamin D and regularly exposing your skin to natural sunlight just might be one of the remedies you need to overcoming chronic pain.

- Avocados. They are rich in heart-healthy mono-unsaturated fatty acids. Along with their many nutrients and polyphenols, avocados are a must-have for an anti-inflammatory diet.
- Carrots. They contain beta-carotene which your body needs to convert to vitamin A, a powerful antioxidant with anti-inflammatory properties. An extra bonus: carrots also contain lutein and zeaxanthine which are important for health of your eyes.
- Dry beans. Navy beans, kidney beans and black beans have many minerals, B-complex vitamins, protein and fiber. The protein and fiber can keep you feeling full longer on fewer calories, and help you drop extra pounds, if you need to lose weight. Maintaining a healthy weight is important for people with any form of arthritis because you will have less pressure on the weight-bearing joints. It also reduces the

inflammation in your body that is a byproduct of body fat. Beans also contain polyphenols that work as antioxidants. Beans are excellent anti-inflammatory in addition to their multiple health benefits.

- Oranges. This very common fruit is an excellent source of vitamin C, potassium, fiber, calcium and folate. Vitamin C is very important for our immune system, strong connective tissues and healthy blood vessels. An antioxidant called beta-cryptoxanthine, found in oranges and other citrus fruits and vegetables like sweet potatoes and cantaloupes, has been found to help reduce the risk of inflammatory conditions in rheumatoid arthritis. Eating oranges should be part of an anti-inflammatory diet, especially if you are suffering from joint pain.

- Sweet potatoes. Along with their purple counterparts, they are rich in vitamin and minerals. Like most colored vegetables, they ar high in vitamin A and carotene, which are powerful antioxidants. Along with their vitamin C and fiber, they are excellent anti-inflammatory foods. In a study from Washington State University, the researchers found that men had reduced markers of inflammation after eating purple potatoes daily for six weeks.

- Green tea. If more people drink tea instead of soda, our nation will be much healthier. The flavonoids in green tea are strong, natural anti-inflammatory compounds that have been shown in many studies to boost the immune system, promote relaxation and reduce stress, along with its other health benefits.

- Papaya and pineapples. They contain enzymes, papain and bromelain, respectively, which have been shown as effective as NSAIDs for pain relief and inflammation.

- Mangoes. This tropical fruit is, not only nutrient-packed, but also a powerful inflammation fighter. In addition to its anti-inflammatory benefits, mangoes are a good source of over 20 vitamins and minerals including vitamin A, C, B6, folate and potassium.

- Coffee. More and more health benefits are being discovered in the caffeine of coffee, as long as you drink it in moderation and have no intolerance or allergy to it. Research suggests caffeine can reduce pain in those suffering from exercise-induced muscular injury and soreness. Not only that, when taken with a standard dose of pain reliever (ibuprofen, for example), one study found that a cup of coffee potentiates the analgesic effects of NSAIDs.

- Grapefruits. They contain a lot of antioxidants which help reduce tissue damages. The high dose of vitamin C, as in oranges, can help decrease the wear and tear on your joints.

- Thyme. It is a herb used in cooking to enhance the flavor of may foods. Research suggests that compounds in thyme may interfere with the perception of pain. Lab studies have shown thyme is as effective as the anti-inflammatory drug, dexamethasone, in reducing pain perception in mice. Despite the lack of conclusive data at this time, it does not hurt to add thyme to your stews, sauces and other dishes for possible pain-free flavor.

- Cloves. It contains an anti-inflammatory chemical called eugenol, which has been shown to inhibit COX-2, a protein that promotes inflammation. This is the same protein that the so-called Cox-2 inhibitor drug such as Celebrex quashes. It is also rich in antioxidants; the combination of its antioxidant and anti-inflammatory properties provide many health benefits from protecting against heart disease to helping stave off cancer, as well as slowing the damage of cartilage and bone caused by arthritis.

- Arnica gel. One study of 204 patients with osteoarthritis in their hands found that using arnica gel for twenty-one days worked just as well at reducing pain as ibuprofen. You can also use it on bruises and sore muscles, replacing pain medications.

- Willow bark. It has been for thousands of years in many different cultures to reduce fever, inflammation and pain. Willow bark is a strong painkilling herb that is still used today to treat back pain, arthritis, headaches, and inflammatory conditions like bursitis and tendinitis. The active ingredient in this herb, salicin, is actually the compound that was first used in the 1800s to develop aspirin. Though it does not work as fast as aspirin, willow bark can provide longer-lasting benefits without the harmful side effects.

Many adults suffer from osteoarthritis (OA), also called degenerative joint disease (DJD), which is a very common painful condition. It is the most common cause of joint pain, affecting millions of Americans. In fact, many of the patients with OA require prescription painkillers or opioid analgesics in order to be active and functioning in their activities of daily living to achieve some quality of life. In my practice, the patients could not tolerate ANSAIDs, which inherently have some dangerous side effects such as gastrointestinal bleed, increased risk of cardiovascular disease and problems for the kidneys and liver from long term use.

Statistically, there are far more deaths from the use of NSAIDs, both over-the-counter and prescriptions, than lethal overdose of narcotic painkillers. If you have some concern about narcotic painkillers that you need for your pain, I advise you to pursue an ' anti-inflammatory diet ', try some alternative therapies as already outlined in this book, and supplement your diet with glucosamine. You may surprise yourself and find yourself less dependent on the narcotic analgesics for pain relief.

In the U.S., glucosamine is one of the most common non-vitamin, non-mineral, dietary supplements used by adults nowadays. Glucosamine is naturally occurring in the shells of shellfish, animal bones and bone marrow, and fungi. It is an amino sugar and a precursor in the biochemical synthesis of glycosylated proteins and lipids. It is marketed to support the structure and function of joints in people suffering from OA.

One research on glucosamine is surprising. A three-year study of glucosamine alone in the form of glucosamine sulfate at 1500mg per day appeared to have a significant benefit in preventing the loss of joint space in the knees of adults with osteoarthritis, resulting in reduction of inflammation and pain.

However, the effectiveness of glucosamine has not been scientifically and conclusively established, and the supplement has been shown to cause harm in high doses, when taken more than 1,500mg daily over time. Since pain is such a personal feeling, if you get relief from glucosamine supplements, you need to be more proactive and learn about possible adverse reactions from it, especially at doses higher than 1,500mg a day. Consult your physician before starting the supplement.

Patients with uncontrolled or intractable chronic pain tend to have elevated levels of cortisol from the adrenal gland, resulting in high cholesterol, lipid and glucose levels, which are almost universal in patients with uncontrolled, intractable pain. High intake of protein with carbohydrate restriction will help control the lipid and glucose levels.

Based on the considerable scientific information and clinical observation in recent years, patients with chronic pain, particularly those requiring opioid treatment, need to have a diet with high protein intake.

Why is protein so critical in patients with chronic pain? There are four sound, theoretical reasons, according to an article by Dr. Forest Tennant, MD, DrPH, published in the Practical Pain Management magazine:

- Endogenous pain relievers are protein derivatives. In the intestine, all protein break down into component parts, which include about two dozen amino acids. There are eight essential amino acids that the body cannot make, and therefore must be suppled through one's diet. In alphabetical order, these are isoleucine, leucine, lysine, methionine, phenylalanine, threonine, tryptophan, and valine. With adequate nutrition, the body can make the other amino acids, with the possible exception of carnitine. Amino acids enter the blood from the intestine and travel to locations in the liver, glands and brain, where they are building blocks for compounds critical for pain relief. These include endorphin, dopamine, serotonin, and gamma aminobutyric acid (GABA). Insulin and thyroid hormones are derived from amino acids. The universal complaint of weakness by patients with severe pain may have many causes, but the lack of protein has to be one of them. Even the receptors to which pain-modulating neurotransmitters (endorphin, serotonin, and GABA) attach are protein moieties. Although no one knows how much protein a patient with pain must take in to provide enough amino acid substrate for the production of these pain-controlling compounds, chances are that it is often not enough.

- Protein builds muscle and cartilage. A number of amino acids are required to build muscle. The amino acid proline is the major building block of collagen, essential for the development of cartilage and inter-vertebral discs.
- Protein activates glucagon. Glucagon is secreted by the liver in response to protein ingestion. Glucagon increases blood glucose levels, and is the only hormone that blocks glucose storage as fat. Eating protein with every meal and every time sugar and starches are eaten will prevent a rapid rise in insulin, storage of any excess glucose as fat, and hypoglycemia that results in carbohydrate cravings and possible pain flare.
- Protein decreases inflammation. Many foods that contain protein, such as fish and green vegetables, contain anti-inflammatory agents.

In a nutshell, patients with chronic pain need a high-protein diet, and do not eat or drink carbohydrates without eating protein at the same time. You can get your protein from nuts, seeds and beans, vegetables, fish, eggs and skinless poultry without the fatty red meat. The trick is eating whole foods as close to their natural state as possible. The more processing a food goes through, the more likely its nutrients, including proteins will be altered or stripped.

A special note:

Good nutrition and a healthy lifestyle are particularly important for people with chronic pain. According to research, smoking is the root cause of many musculoskeletal disorders. Smoking can cause changes in pain processing and perception. Epidemiologically, smokers have more pain, increased pain frequency, an increased number of pain sites, increased low back pain, and most importantly, an increased incidence of disabling low back pain. Pathophysiologically, smokers are more prone to disc degeneration, have impaired healing and pain pathways. Thus, smokers take longer to heal. Therefore, in order to maximize the effectiveness of pain management, patients with chronic pain are advised to stop smoking.

DO NOT ADD INSULT TO INJURY!

Chapter Twelve

Closing summary

As a pain doctor, trained to relieve patient's pain at the best of your ability, you owe it to your patients to help control their pain and take steps to help them function with some quality of life and dignity. If the only way to accomplish those goals is to prescribe controlled substances, when other modalities failed or not available, you should not hesitate to do so. If it becomes apparent to you that a patient wishes to choose a course of treatment that is not consistent with appropriate medical care, you must not yield to the patients' desire.

No recognized standard of care exists for prescribing controlled substances for chronic pain, but it certainly is acceptable when the medications are prescribed to control and reduce pain, alleviate anxiety, avoid worsening of depression, or improve the quality of sleep. Indeed, withholding these drugs when necessary could well constitute inappropriate care. The greatest risk for the prescribing practitioner is falling into the trap of being duped by drug-seeking or drug-abusing patients. Unfortunately, there is no foolproof process to demonstrate the legitimacy of a pain patient. And it is over-reaching and inappropriate to expect the prescribing doctors to serve as police or detective.

The word ' drug ' has such a bad, terrifying connotation. In our federal system here in the U.S., it is such a big net, encompassing marijuana, dangerous street heroin and cocaine, and prescription opioids for pain by licensed physicians. Under the Law, the prescribing physicians are automatically treated as drug dealers and distributors. This is so absurd!

Another thing that is so ridiculous and unfair in the victimization of physicians is the legal phrase of ' prescribe and dispense '. The legal language is supposed to be very specific, and even the act of murder has several different degrees and forms. Many attorneys are good at ' splitting the hair ', and have won cases.

When I received my 83 counts of indictment on May 15, 2013, I was very bewildered by the charges of prescribing and dispensing controlled substances illegally even though I had never dispensed any controlled substances from my two offices. In the distant past, there might be a few doctors dispensing some Tylenol #3 or Vicodin tablets from their offices; given the liabilities and the antagonistic, witch-hunting law enforcement agencies in the past decade, I am not aware of any doctors willing to keep and dispense controlled substances on their premises.

In order to prescribe any medications, physicians usually go through patient's history, brief or comprehensive, and perform a physical examination, brief or comprehensive, form a clinical diagnosis before prescribing. By definition, dispensing is to supply medicine according to a prescription, usually by a professional, licensed pharmacist. They are two separate, independent professionals involved before a patient receives the medication. Both the physician and pharmacist had to go through considerable education and training to do their jobs, and these are two different acts with separate responsibilities and liabilities. Unfortunately and unfairly, the prescribing pain doctors have to bear the two burdens under the law which makes no distinction between prescribing and dispensing, while the dispensing pharmacists are generally exempt from any legal liability, especially when they are willing to collaborate and collude with the investigating authorities to ' put the doctor on the cross '.

In the U.S., we have been fighting the ' war on drugs ' for several decades, and the problem does not seem to be getting better with more and more arrests and overdose deaths. The government feels discouraged and frustrated, and many of its officials are trying to find scapegoats to blame and to reach a quick resolution. There is no question that prescriptions for Oxycontin, Hydrocodone and Methadone have soared in recent years. It is also clear that there are a few ' bad ' doctors and pill mills who unscrupulously hand out prescriptions for painkillers to patients who should not get them, and to drug addicts and drug dealers pretending to be pain patients. But it is far from certain that the drug abuse and overdoses are as dire as the government is making it to be.

More problems are created due to a decade of aggressive policing, obstinate federal law enforcement agencies, the encroachment of law enforcement into the private practice of medicine, and lax government oversight. The DEA, in particular, has been scaring reputable, well-intended and conscientious doctors away from pain management since 1990s.

Many people agree but afraid to express their opinion that the government has been waging an aggressive, intemperate, unjustified and over-powering war on pain doctors, who are soft and easy targets. One patient told the Village Voice, " you worry every day that medicines won't be available for much longer, or your doctor won't be there tomorrow because he or she has been arrested by the DEA ". Many medical schools now advise their students not to choose pain management as a career because the field is too fraught with potential legal dangers.

We must stop threatening the prescribing pain doctors with expensive (actually cost-prohibitive), stressful, frivolous and damaging charges of diversion, abuse and/or illegal prescriptions for controlled substances. More efforts should be directed to combat the theft of drugs from homes, hospitals, warehouses, manufacturing facilities, pharmacies and en route to and from pharmacies. The DEA, DOJ, Congress and state and local authorities should end the senseless persecution of doctors in pain management and allow them to pursue whatever treatment options they feel are in the best interests of their patients, free from the watchful eye and broad net of law enforcement. It is everyone's job to have an open mind, to get educated and to educate others for better understanding of our problems.

PATIENTS WITH CHRONIC, UNBEARABLE PAIN DESERVE TREATMENTS, NOT LABELS!

More and more people, not just in the U.S., are suffering from chronic, severe pain, and the need for public outcry around the needs of Americans with chronic, painful conditions is greater today than ever before in light of the multi-front assault occurring daily on your right of dignified, impartial, compassionate care. In this era of rising number of deaths involving opioid painkillers and heroin, regulators and many doctors are restricting access to drugs like Oxycontin and Hydrocodone. With the pendulum swinging to the other direction, many patients who genuinely need the medications to manage their pain say they are being left behind, neglected, minimized and ostracized.

In a December 9, 2016 CNN report, fentanyl abuse was the primary reason for the 73% rise of overdose deaths from synthetic opioids, according to the estimates by CDC. Investigations by the CDC showed that the fentanyl involved in those 2015 overdose deaths was not from prescription medications containing fentanyl, it was from Fentanyl illegally manufactured. According to the DEA reports, they seized a record of 167 kilograms of illicit fentanyl in 2015.

Fentanyl is at least 100 times stronger than morphine, and at least 30 times more powerful than heroin. I think, part of the problem is because too many people were unable to get prescription opioids for effective pain treatment.

Even doctors face predicaments and some can't agree on how to help their pain patients. Very sadly, I am seeing a ' civil war ' developing timidly in the pain community. It reminds me of a McCarthyism that is silencing so many people who are simply scared. Dr. Sean Mackey, who oversees the renowned pain management program of Stanford University, said, " The thing is, we all want black and white. We don't do well with nuance. And this is an incredibly nuanced issue."

The fact is neither side has much evidence about the benefits or consequences of long-term use of opioids because almost no such studies exist. The risks of long-term opioid therapy are important to be recognized and more education is needed. How about thousands and thousands of people who die every year from anti-inflammatory, non-steroidal medications like ibuprofen? Nobody seems to be talking about that.

The personal experiences of patients living with pain and seeking empathy and medical care are often against the odds. Misguided and politically motivated state and federal policies are impeding access to appropriate and reasonable medical care for people struggling with chronic pain and deterring even the most caring medical providers from treating patients with chronic pain. It is therefore imperative that people suffering from chronic pain, including our veterans, raise their voices together and singularly to demand the care you deserve. It is only by casting your vote, in our country of democracy, and continuing to demand attention to the ever-worsening barriers, prejudicial apathy and unacceptable suffering that change will occur!

We do not want pill mills and unconscionable doctors, which are very few in numbers, and definitely a problem, but the reaction to them is not only excessive, it over-shoots its intended target. Undoubtedly, all well-intended, legitimate doctors want to stop drug diversion and abuse and to close down all pill mills, if possible by our government's law enforcement, that are violating good medical practice principles, endangering and stigmatizing healthcare providers. The over-aggressive, unreasonable restrictions by the DEA are costing the majority of legitimate patients and doctors much grief, frustration, fear, time, energy, discomfort and distress.

We must view this entire picture through the lens that patients come first --- what they need for their medical problems. How to get the system of our government to respond in the way remains a frustrating problem. Just because there are a few out there that abuse prescription pain medications, that does not mean everyone suffering from chronic pain should be punished!

Diversion and abuse are real and of significance; the doctors agree and understand. However, the government's short-sighted efforts to quickly solve those problems may end up causing an enduring public health crisis of extraordinary proportions with significant economic impact. When it comes to deadliness, no single substance comes close to tobacco. To put its risk in perspective, more Americans die from tobacco-caused health problems like lung cancer and heart disease than from reported drug overdoses, car accidents and homicides combined. Overall, cigarette smoking is linked to one in five deaths in the U.S. each year, according to CDC estimates. Nearly 42,000 of the total 480,000 deaths every year from smoking are caused by second-hand smoke.

The drug problems in our American society are very complicated, more so than other countries. I think we must look at it with a multi-faceted approach and from different perspectives. Every member of our society needs to be involved because the drug problem has reached all levels of the American society, poor and rich, men and women, blue-colored workers, professionals, street-peddlers, children, youths and adults, private sectors and government (local, state and federal).

It is my opinion that the biggest barrier to effective pain treatment, at this time, continues to be bad public policy. Please let me remind everyone that those patients who end up on opioid pain management have usually tried everything else unsuccessfully.

Special note:

Patients who are prescribed and need multiple opioids to control their pain should be given blood toxicology at regular intervals, in addition to urine drug tests, to determine and ascertain the hemodynamic steady-state. Typically, the therapeutic windows for opioids are narrow, but patients with chronic pain tend to have higher therapeutic levels of the medications due to tolerance. Despite the higher doses of opioids, many patients were found to be able to function normally, working with satisfactory performance as a contributing member of society, enjoying quality of sleep, having normal relationship with loved ones, and showing no cognitive impairment.

When deadly accidents happened to these patients who need higher doses of opioids to live, medical examiners instinctively and conveniently certified the death certificates with poly-pharmacy even though other factors, with careful and responsible investigations, were involved. This irresponsible diagnosis of poly-pharmacy on the death certificate of your patient could potentially bring the pain doctor a lot of legal problems. Therefore, a drug test using the blood when your patient is medically stable and functional while on opioids is one piece of very important, medical information for your patient's file, because it will prove that your prescriptions did not cause your patient's death.

This is also important for families and spouses whose loved ones with life insurance coverage might have been killed in motor vehicle accidents. Accidental death in a motor vehicle accident is usually covered by the life insurance company, NOT ' drug overdose '. The diagnosis of poly-pharmacy by the medical examiner or coroner might not be correct and it is used by insurance companies to deny benefits. If your loved one was functioning normally in his or her activities of daily living while taking opioids prescribed by the doctor before the tragic car accident without any aberrant behavior or non-compliance, you have a legitimate case to pursue insurance benefits.

If your loved one is suffering from chronic pain, you need to be proactive and interested in educating yourself about the pain conditions he or she is facing. Show your suffering loved one that you care and work with the treating physician. Patients with chronic pain face a long, bumpy road in their struggle, and understanding and support from their family and loved ones are imperative.

Addendum

There were eighty-three counts against me in the federal indictment, charging that the controlled substances for pain were prescribed without legitimate medical purposes. The 83 counts came from a total of ten patients out of the hundreds, if not thousands, of patients I saw over the years. Three of those ten patients were under-cover DEA agents, posing as patients with audio-visual wire-tapping. I would like my readers to know the conditions and treatments of those patients with my brief summary for each of them below and make your own informed judgment. The judge never had a chance to hear in court or review the following patients' clinical information because, with the advice of my public defender and the lack of resources, I had to make a plea agreement to one of the 83 counts, admitting that I prescribed the controlled substance, Hydrocodone, without legitimate medical purposes to one undercover agent.

Patient #1:

It was a 46 years old male who was under my care for over ten years for migraine, chronic low back pain and panic disorder. The major cause for his anxiety and panic disorder was his painful marital problems and legal custody issues about his daughter. These situations caused him a great deal of stress, which aggravated his panic disorder and chronic pain.

He was a frequent user of the emergency room at CGH Medical Center in Sterling, Illinois; Most of his ER visits involved severe headaches with nausea and vomiting; others were presented with complaints of low back pain. ER doctors ordered CT scan and MRI of his head quite a few .times. He was also seen at the ER on many occasions for acute anxiety and panic attacks, leading to chest pain and shortness of breath.

His back surgery, lumbar laminectomy, had not given him any relief for his low back pain. Over 50% of patients with neck and back pain had to resort to medical pain management with opioids after surgeries due to Failed Neck and Back Surgery Syndrome, in order to gain some satisfactory level of ADL (activities of daily living), to improve functionality and quality of life.

The medications of NORCO and Xanax I prescribed were medically necessary and appropriate for this patient, and were within the therapeutic dosage ranges, as shown in his office notes. Patient was well-tolerant of opioid analgesics due to his long history of therapeutic treatment for his chronic pain with opioids by other doctors before he came under my care. In fact, he had taken opioid analgesics much more potent than NORCO prescribed by other doctors such as Fentanyl patches.

I learnt from patient's mother that he passed away during his driving trip to New York for a job, with three other co-workers in the car.

His diagnoses included:

- Chronic low back pain
- Long history of intractable headaches (migraine, diagnosed by his neurologist)
- Anxiety/Panic Disorder
- Failed back surgery syndrome
- History of hypertension

Patient #2:

This 40 years old female patient had suffered from chronic low back pain and other pain conditions for over seven years with opioid treatments prior to becoming my patient. Thus, she was not opioid-naïve, and her tolerance to opioids was expected. She also had on-going psychiatric and psychological treatments at the local hospital, and received prescriptions for anxiety and depression.

She seemed to have suffered a lot of stress and anxiety with her family problems, especially the loss of custody for her children and other domestic issues. The prescription Xanax helped her deal with the mental health issues. For pain management, she was prescribed NORCO 10/325, one tablet every 8 hours as needed orally, well within the recommended dosage. I also prescribed Ibuprofen for her. Due to her mental health issues, I was very careful in prescribing painkillers for her, limiting to only one opioid analgesic. She was also ordered and given alternative treatments for her pain which included therapeutic massages, physical therapy with ultrasound, and TENS to be used at home. She was also referred to orthopedic specialist due to her diagnosis of lumbar disc herniation, and the orthopedic specialist performed epidural injections for her pain.

She reported, at least, an 8 on a scale of 10 for her pain most of the time. At the time of her death, she was found to have a few other medications not prescribed by me, and these included Methadone, amitriptyline, Valproic acid, nortriptyline, acetaminophen and diphenhydramine (Tylenol-PM) in dosages many times over the recommended ranges. As an OTC medication, the recommended dose for Tylenol-PM is no more than two tablets in a 24-hour period because of potentially dangerous side effects with the anti-histamine. One of the more serious and significant side effects is cognitive impairment, such as dementia or delirium, identified as confusion.

Her diagnoses included:

• Chronic, intractable low back pain
• Lumbar disc herniation, L5-S1.
• Status post motor vehicle accident X 2 or more
• Frequent headaches
• Status post multiple injuries such as a fall from a bicycle

- History of depression with anxiety
- History of ADHD

Her mother was also my patient for chronic pain, and informed me that the Sherriff found a bottle of Tylenol-PM almost empty by the deceased patient's body.

Patient #3:

This 46 years of male patient of mine sustained a major injury to his head, neck and back after a fall from a flight of stairs. He suffered from low back pain for a long time prior to his visit to my office, with multiple MRIs. He also suffered from right knee pain and received treatments from orthopedic including arthroscopy.

He also received care from anesthesiologist/pain specialist and underwent several percutaneous steroid injections for three of his lumbar vertebral joints. The same doctor prescribed Duragesic, a brand for the very potent analgesic, fentanyl, due to his persistent, severe pain. Patient also received epidural injection with anesthesia by the same pain specialist/anesthesiologist.

He also had tried NORCO and Vicodin prescribed by three other healthcare providers without satisfactory pain relief. Due to his long, complex chronic pain history, it was my professional judgment to start him on Morphine Sulfate-ER (the extended release form) and NORCO 10/325 to manage his pain. He responded well to the treatment regimen I prescribed; in fact, he was well enough to travel out of town for jobs which involved physical work and labor.

I tried to change the MS-ER to Embeda, which was a new long-acting morphine product with very minimal abuse potential (a new abuse-deterrent formulation at the time). Unfortunately, Embeda was cost-prohibitive for him and there was no generic substitution for it at the time. Over the course of his pain management, some changes were made with the medications, which was not unusual in pain practice.

His diagnoses included:

- Failed back surgery syndrome
- Chronic headaches, post-traumatic
- Chronic knee pain
- Lumbar disc disease with right radiculopathy
- Multiple injuries secondary to falls
- Struggle with his spouse regarding his chronic pain with little understanding about his suffering

Patient #4:

This 51 years old female patient presented with chronic pain in her low back, left hip, and crampy abdominal pain, especially during bowel movements. She rated her overall pain a ' 6 ' on a scale of 10. In her Pain Outcome Profile, the pain sometimes interfered with her ability to walk, to climb stairs and to bathe herself. She also stated that prolonged sitting increased her back pain. The pain also disrupted her sleep and made her depressed and affected her self-esteem. Other significant medical history included injuries to her sacral area at least three times with fractures. She sustained a four-wheeler accident resulting in multiple fractures of ribs. Her pain was further complicated and aggravated by a motor vehicle accident in November of 2010.

Since she had tried NORCO in the past with little relief of pain, I started her on low-dose Methadone along with Elavil 10mg at bedtime. Methadone is an effective opioid analgesic, inexpensive with low addictive potential. It is not known to cause euphoria. She had no contra-indication for its use. A NSAID of Mobic was added. I prescribed NORCO later for her break-through pain; probably due to tolerance, I changed it to fast-acting oxycondone-IR, as needed for break-through pain. She seemed to be doing well after oxycodone-IR was added, and I was able to decrease her Methadone dose from 60mg to 40mg a day.

Due to the persistent complaint of pain in her left hip, I ordered an MRI. I even contacted a privately-owned MRI facility for a reduced price for her MRI to make it affordable for her. Due to inconsistency of her urinary drug tests more than once and her non-compliance with the MRI order, I had to discharge her from my care for possible diversion of controlled substances.

Her diagnoses included:

- Chronic low back pain
- Internal derangement of left knee
- Arthropathy of left hip
- Status-post vehicular accidents (4-wheeler and automobile)
- Post-traumatic fractures of ribs and sacrum

Patient #5:

This was a 54 years old male who sustained a motor vehicle accident in 2001 with multiple injuries. He sustained another injury while lifting something heavy in 2005; he was treated by orthopedic surgeon after the lifting injury of her low back with potent opioid analgesics such as Dilaudid, NORCO, and Fentanyl patches, in addition to a series of epidural steroid injections.

His initial office visit with me was on 09/06/2008 with complaints of persistent neck and back pain. With his complex and long history of opioid treatment for chronic pain, I started him on Suboxone and Mobic (both are non-addicting with analgesic properties). On 5/20/2009, he had an abnormal MRI showing multiple disc herniations in both the cervical and lumbar spine. To achieve better pain control, the Suboxone was discontinued and replaced by Dilaudid 4mg, every 4 to 6 hours as needed, I also prescribed low-dose Xanax for his anxiety and insomnia.

I added longer-acting Methadone later, hoping for better pain coverage. Patient did have improvement with the regimen. Unfortunately, his UDTs showed repeated inconsistencies, and other medications NOT prescribed by me; I discharged him from my care on 08/11/2011. Dealing with and treating patients with chronic, intractable can be and is challenging all the time, and frustrating sometimes.

His diagnoses included:

- Chronic pain secondary multiple MVAs
- Multiple cervical disc herniations
- Multiple lumbar disc herniations
- Degenerative disease of the spine
- Spinal stenosis
- Chronic headaches
- Anxiety with insomnia
- Status-post surgery of the left shoulder with rotator cuff dysfunction
- Refractory chronic pain syndrome

Patient #6

This 43 years old male patient sustained a severe crush injury to his left hand at work in 2009 and was seen by me for the first time on 03/17/2009. He was a machine operator at a printing shop when a 750-ton power press landed on his left hand. Significant history included opioid treatment for his pain and sedatives for anxiety and sleep.

He had two reconstructive surgeries for his left hand at a teaching hospital. His initial complaint was severe pain in his left hand. Patient later sustained a severe painful injury to his left leg with his entire left foot grossly bent and twisted with marked swelling and painful movements. He was walking with crutches, walker and cane for quite some time.

Due to his past history with opioid treatment of pain, I started him with Dilaudid 4mg, every six hours as needed. I also prescribed low-dose Xanax for his anxiety and insomnia, which was medically necessary and appropriate. He rated the pain in his left leg ' 10 ' on a scale of 10. The pain affected his mental health with increasing anxiety and some depression. It was medically necessary for me to increase his Xanax to 2mg every 8 hours as needed. For better pain control, I added long-acting Methadone 10mg, every 8 hours. While under my care, he continued his physical therapy and follow-up with his orthopedic surgeon. He was also consulted by pain specialist/anesthesiologist for pain management in 2011.

He tolerated his medications well and was able to function without any cognitive impairment.

His diagnoses included:

- Pain secondary to severe crush injury of left hand
- Status-post reconstructive surgeries of left hand
- Severe pain secondary to significant injury to the left leg with deformity
- Neuralgia of left leg
- Severe pain secondary peri-rectal abscess
- Chronic pain syndrome

Patient #7:

It was a 55 years old female patient who presented to my office as a new patient with many years of chronic pain. She was approved for medical disability with Medicare since 1994 due to a diagnosis of multiple sclerosis. Pain can be one of the worst manifestations of MS; the National Multiple Sclerosis Society estimates that up to 50% of MS patients are plagued by chronic pain.

She had all necessary workup for her different pain, including x-rays of the spine, CT and MRI of the head ordered by neurologist, and pelvic ultrasound for her complaints of lower abdominal and pelvic pain. Besides opioid painkillers such as Vicodin-ES and Ultram for her intractable headaches, she also had Hydrocodone for a fracture of her right wrist prescribed by her orthopedic surgeon as well as Restoril for insomnia.

She continued to suffer from chronic pain and came to see me for the first time in December of 2008. With her long history of treatment with opioid analgesics and persistent pain symptom, I started her on a long-acting OxyContin 20mg, every 12 hours, for a trial, while she continued her Vicodin-ES as needed for break-through pain. Due to the nature of her pain conditions with MS and Fibromyalgia, it was not easy to titrate her pain medications in order to achieve the best results of pain management – decrease in pain level, increase in functionality. And improvement of mental health.

Accidental fall is not uncommon due to gait disturbance with MS; she suffered a fracture of her right arm (the bone, humerus) and treated by her orthopedic surgeon. Her fall had nothing to do with the pain medications which tolerated well without any signs of cognitive impairment. In fact, she was doing well with a therapeutic regimen of OxyContin, Dilaudid and Xanax.

Her diagnoses included:

- Multiple Sclerosis
- Intractable migraine
- Pain secondary to fracture of right arm
- Chronic pelvic pain secondary to dyspareunia
- History of uterine endometriosis, diagnosed by her gynecologist
- Insomnia
- Fibromyalgia
- Anxiety with panic disorder
- Chronic pain secondary to history of multiple abdominal surgeries.

Patient #8:

The 48 years old female patient came to see me for the first time on 02/23/2005 due to persistent pain in her neck after injury sustained at work. Even after surgery for her cervical spine, the pain continued to give her a lot of problems including headaches, and painful movements of her neck. Her symptoms were made much worse when she sustained a motor vehicle accident one week after her neck surgery.

Patient was referred to a pain specialist/anesthesiologist by her surgeon; she was prescribed Xanax and Hydrocodone for and underwent several epidural steroid injections as an out-patient at a local hospital near my office. Patient had a few other alternative treatment modalities for pain management, including acupuncture, chiropractic adjustments, therapeutic massages, TENS and ultrasound. She also went through four weeks of rehab exercises for strengthening of muscles and improving RON of joints.

In addition to opioids, I also prescribed Ibuprofen, Arthrotic and Toradol at different times to help her pain. Despite different treatment modalities and medicines, her pain was difficult to control; her personal life and stressful family situations made it very challenging to achieve optimal pain management. She seemed to be accident-prone, including falling down the steps at home in 2006. She was no stranger to the ER of CGH Medical Center in Sterling, Illinois,

We did discuss about discontinuing OxyContin on several occasions and gave Suboxone a try. She did not fill her prescription for Suboxone and requested to stay on OxyContin for some pain relief. Her back pain was getting so aggravated after her brother threw her on the floor that I had to send her to the hospital for MRI of lumbar spine on 04/09/2008. The MRI showed multiple fractures of the right transverse processes from L1 to L4.

Even though the patient had multiple painful conditions with confirmed diagnoses, when she started to show aberrant drug-seeking behavior with different doctors on the PMP reports, I decided to discharge her from my care on 10/23/2009.

Her diagnoses included:

- Cervical disc disease with radiculopathy
- Degenerative joint disease of the spine
- Chronic pain with exacerbation due to multiple injuries at different times

- Status-post multiple MVAs
- History of domestic physical abuse resulting in multiple fractures of lumbar vertebrae
- Chronic pain secondary to bilateral carpal tunnel syndrome. The symptomatology of the right wrist was severe enough to require surgery with transposition of the ulnar nerve at the elbow
- Chronic headaches
- History of ADHD
- Anxiety and panic disorder

It was sad that this patient colluded and collaborated with the government out of spite to file a Victim Statement with the court, trying to place the blame on me for her problems. I tried to help her complicated pain conditions and her problematic life at the best I could with good intention and compassion. This was really an epitome of legal manipulation by the prosecution and twisting of facts and covering up of truth by the misguided patient in the persecution of pain doctors. Today, pain doctors just can't win; you are damned if you do and you are damned if you don't.

Patient #9 (a undercover agent from DEA):

His initial office visit was 03/15/2011 with complaint of pain in his left foot. He further complained of some tingling and numbness sometimes; walking made his pain worse. He admitted to having used narcotic pain medications including OxyContin in the past. He stated in his medical record that he sustained a stress fracture of his left foot during war duties in Iraq. The pain limited his physical activities including his ability to climb stairs. The pain also affected his endurance and strength.

A urinary drug test was done during his initial office visit; it revealed high level of Tramadol (brand name, Ultram). Tramadol is a narcotic pain reliever for moderate and moderately-severe pain. Obviously, the undercover agent posing as patient had been taking

Tramadol for his pain. During his three office visits, I gave orders for x-rays of his left foot, to be followed by MRI.

I started with Voltaren 75mg, twice a day for pain; but his request for Vicodin was reasonable and acceptable considering his history of pain treatment with Ultram and others in the past. The Vicodin was to be taken as needed, and patient was instructed not to use it if the pain did not require medication.

His diagnoses included:

- Post-traumatic injury to the left foot with stress fracture
- Chronic pain with interference with functionality and quality of life
- History of therapeutic pain treatment with Tramadol

Patient #10 (second undercover DEA agent):

According to her self-reporting history, she was involved in a MVA in 2008 and suffered mild non-specific pain which interfered with her ability to walk, to climb stairs and to bathe sometimes. The pain also caused her problem with sleep, and made it hard for her to work as a house-keeper, sweeping, mopping, cleaning windows, etc. She felt considerable pain in her shoulders and back after work.

Her PMP (Prescription Monitoring Program) reports showed that she was treated by other providers for her pain with Hydrocodone (NORCO 10/325) prior to her visits with me. Her urinary drug tests revealed patient to be compliant and consistent with the pain medications prescribed. Even though her physical examination at the office did not reveal any acute changes or neurologic deficits, in my professional judgment, it was acceptable and appropriate to prescribe NOTCO for her based on her complaints of pain, history of MVA, and history of previous treatment with opioids.

It was better and safer, furthermore, for her to obtain legal prescriptions from a physician with proper monitoring an follow-up instead of getting controlled substances from friends.

Her diagnoses: included:

- Chronic pain involving shoulders and back
- Myalgia
- Status-post MVA in 2008 with persistent post-traumatic pain
- History of therapeutic treatment with opioid painkillers

Patient #11 (the third DEA undercover agent):

This male patient presented with complaints of generalized aches after workout; sometimes, the pain made it hard for him to continue his exercise. He had a total of three office visits, about four weeks apart. He specifically requested prescriptions for Oxycodone for his pain, and I told him every visit that his pain was not severe enough to require Oxycondone, which was used for moderate to severe pain. My refusal to give him what he wanted could be heard clearly on the audio tapes in the wiretap he was wearing.

Many practitioners, including dentists, family physicians and emergency room doctors prescribed hydrocodone to be used for pain as needed, every four to six hours. It was my usual practice NOT to give automatic refills for controlled substances, even though the Law allows the refills. It was also my practice to monitor patients regularly and closely with follow-up visits.

His diagnoses included:

1. General myositis and myalgia after workout.

Special note: Most people would agree this was some kind of entrapment with the DEA agents posing as patients suffering from chronic pain, requesting opioid painkillers from caring physicians.

Speaking of opioid painkillers prescribed by dentists, more than half of the drugs prescribed to patients after wisdom tooth extraction surgeries went unused in a recent Drug and Alcohol Dependence study, conducted at the University of Pennsylvania School of Dental Medicine. These pill numbers from oral surgeons and dentists can and do translate to a staggering annual figure: over 100 million opioid pills.

This means they are available for misuse and abuse by patients, their loved ones or others. Many patients keep unused opioids ' for a rainy day ', according to the study. They think that they may need it for pain again, or a family member will need them some day. Our government, federal, state and local, should consider more take-back days for opioids including secured disposal boxes for extra and unused opioid pills.

Despite the so-called opioid epidemic, healthcare providers will continue to prescribe these drugs because people, including those working for the government, will need them for pain. We have a long way to go due to the level of health illiteracy. Everyone needs to be educated at a level they can understand!

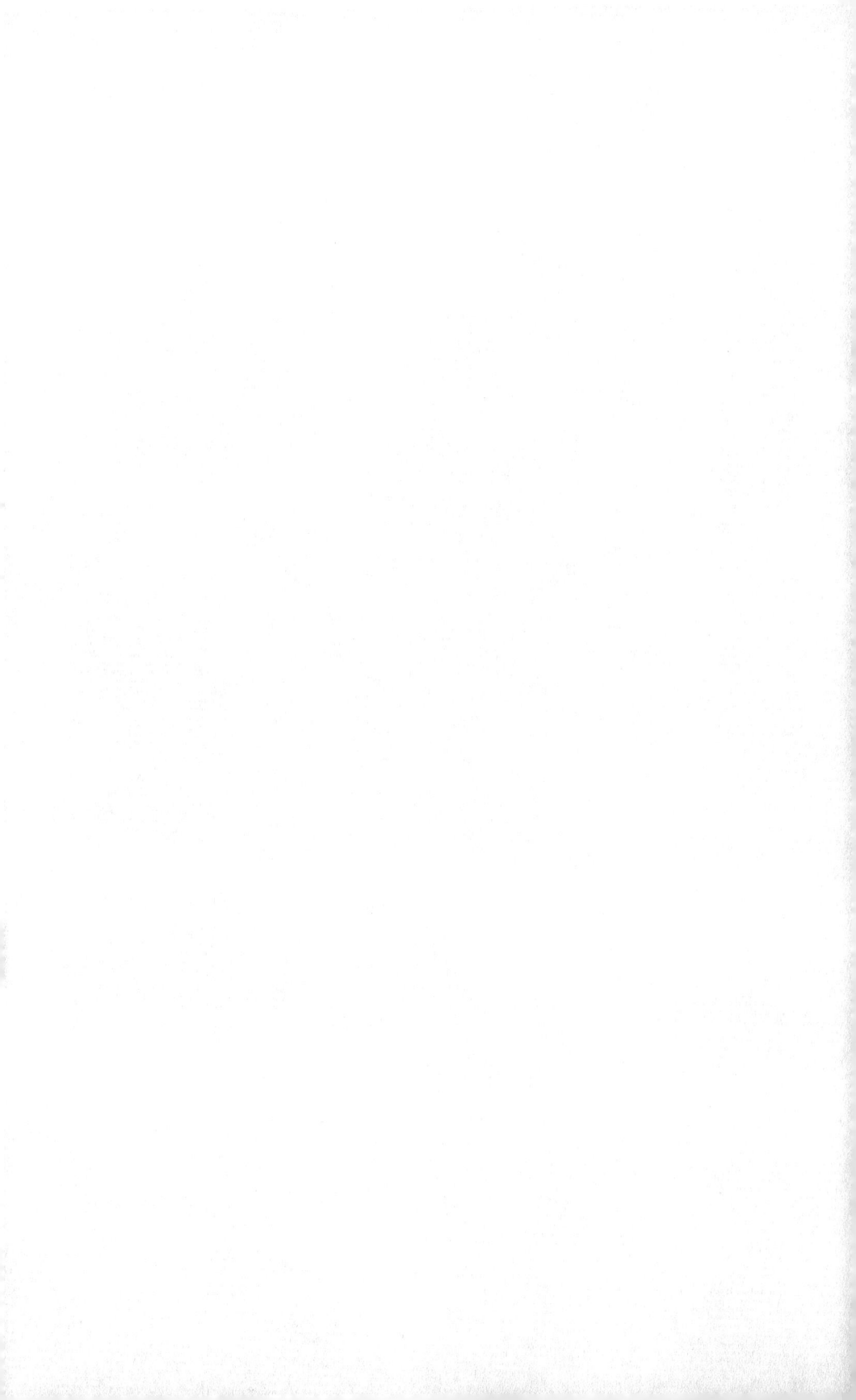

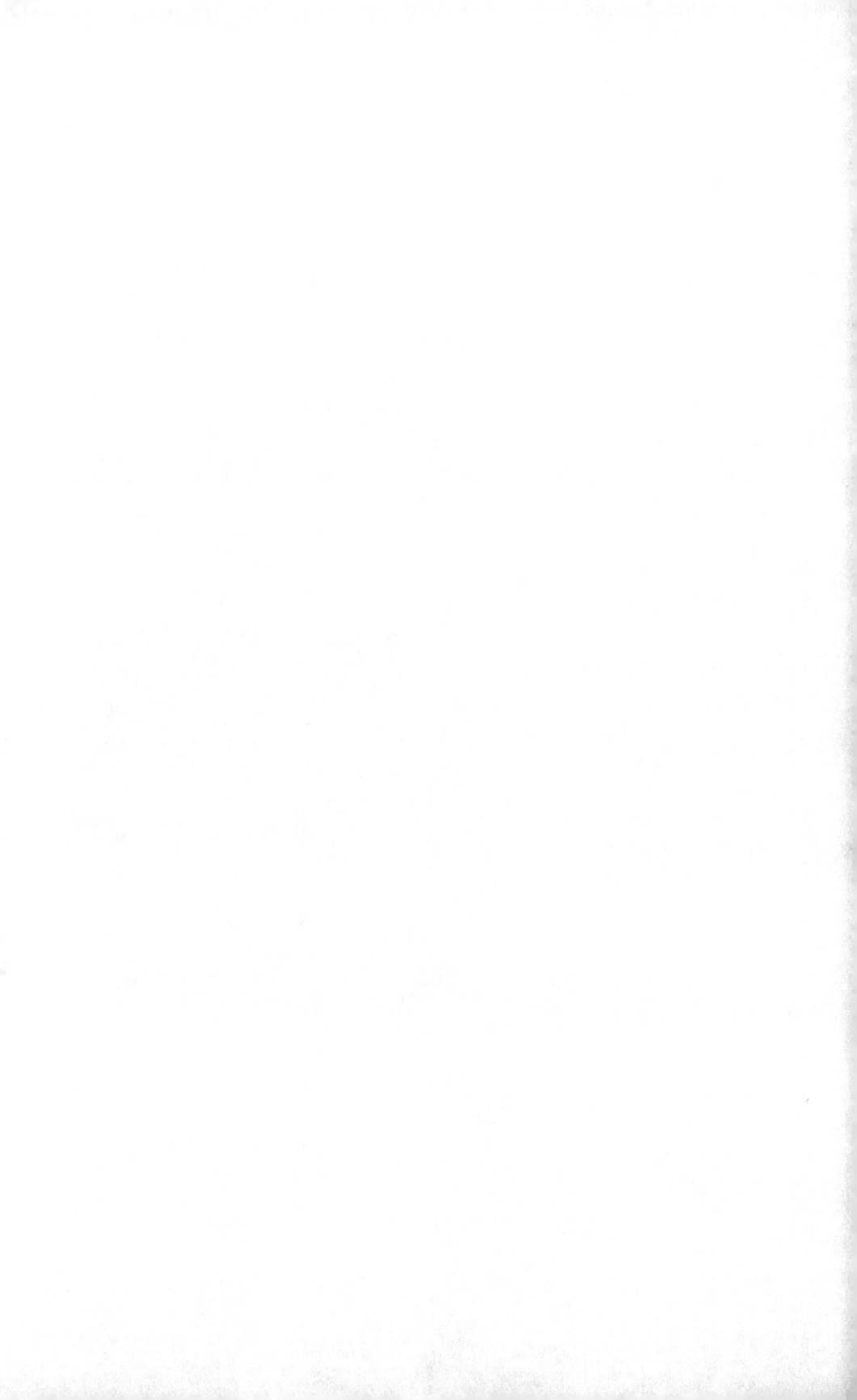